URINE THERAPY

URINE
THERAPY

Nature's Elixir
for
Good Health

FLORA PESCHEK-BÖHMER, PH.D.,
AND GISELA SCHREIBER

TRANSLATED FROM THE GERMAN BY
HANS-GEORG BAKKER

Healing Arts Press
Rochester, Vermont

Healing Arts Press
One Park Street
Rochester, Vermont 05767
www.InnerTraditions.com

Healing Arts Press is a division of Inner Traditions International

Copyright © 1997 by Wilhelm Heyne Verlag GmbH & Co. KG, München

Translation © 1999 by Inner Traditions International

Note to the reader: This book is intended as an informational guide. The remedies, approaches, and techniques described herein are meant to supplement, and not to be a substitute for, professional medical care or treatment. They should not be used to treat a serious ailment without prior consultation with a qualified health care professional.

Library of Congress Cataloging-in-Publication Data

Peschek-Böhmer, Flora.
    [Urin-therapie praxisbuch. English]
    Urine therapy : nature's elixir for good health / Flora Peschek-Böhmer and Gisela Schreiber.
       p.   cm.
    ISBN 978-089281-799-3
    1. Urine—Therapeutic use. I. Schreiber, Gisela. II. Title.
RM298.U7P4713   1999
615'.36—dc21   99-18418
                               CIP

Printed and bound in Canada

10 9 8 7 6 5 4

Text design and layout by Jenna Dixon
This book was typeset in Sabon, with display type in Trajan.

CONTENTS

PREFACE

Finally, nobody says "yuck" anymore

When I started writing a book about a rarely discussed topic like urine, I was prepared to break taboos and fight against excessive hygiene education. The reactions of my readers to my first book, *Urine therapy—a taboo gets broken,* and my daily experiences in my naturopathic office in Hamburg-Winterhude proved me right to an astonishing degree. A lot has changed since that first book was published in 1995. I cannot be as proud about the growing climate of acceptance as you, the readers, who dared to try out a new and different way. To rely on yourself for healing, rather than on medications, means to take an active role in your own health care, rather than remaining in the role of a victim.

Try talking with your friends and relatives about urine therapy. You will be surprised how many of them already know about it or even have tried it. However, you will probably meet with resistance, as well. It is never easy to reverse decades of old prejudice. The small child who has just learned to leave the diaper behind receives praise for using the potty. But if the child tries to reach into the pot, he or she will be told "Pee is yucky." Later the child will be taught to shut the bathroom door, to wash his or her hands thoroughly, and to leave the table with an "excuse me" rather than with an "I got to go." Mention of the body's excretions is taboo, acceptable only in the medical office. Grandpa's advice for fighting athlete's foot, "Just pee on your feet in the shower," makes him a screwball. If one would try it out, though, one would realize that Grandpa is right. Urine is a universal tool for the body to be used internally and externally, as well as in the household. In the extreme case, it can even save lives (shipwrecked passengers or victims of natural catastrophes have often been saved from dying of thirst by drinking their own urine).

In this book my coauthor and I collected the experiences of my readers and patients and my own experiences as a therapist. It should serve the practice even more than the first book. Use it as a resource book and trust yourself to be right.

Flora Peschek-Böhmer

CONVERSATIONS WITH MY PATIENTS

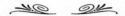

We talk openly about the "private place"

> **Peter K., 47, auto mechanic,** looked at me with big eyes: "Drink my own urine? I am not going to do that. That's disgusting!" Four weeks later the same patient stood in front of me smiling: "For a week I've drunk a glass of my urine every morning. I feel great!" In between came many talks with me and a lot of courage from him—a courage that has been rewarded.

The things taught by mother need to be overcome. "Pee is yucky" say the grown-ups, when the small child examines the liquid in the potty with his or her hands. Later on in life all our experience with toilets is associated with a certain embarrassment. Public bathrooms often smell bad and are dirty. Urine becomes a taboo. In a restaurant we "excuse" ourselves, use the "bath" room, or "put some more makeup on." If somebody got up from the table declaring "I have to urinate," everyone would be embarrassed.

Over the years that I have used urine therapy I have learned how to gently dismantle my patients' inhibitions about their own bodily fluid. One thing never seems to change: when I propose this therapy for the first time, most of my patients reply "I could never do this." I counter by telling them about all the other patients of mine who gave me the same answer and now drink a glass of urine every morning. And I talk about the beneficial physical changes that were brought about through urine therapy.

> **Margaret P., massage therapist,** suffered for years from hay fever and various food allergies. Without medications, sometimes even cortisone injections, she could not control her ailments. She heard about urine therapy, read my first book on the subject, and made her first attempts: "The first morning I left the urine in the glass until it was cooler (about 10 minutes) and took my cup of coffee with me into the bathroom. Then I drank a sip of the urine, which was indeed without an odor. Honestly: I started gagging right away. This was not because of the taste—which, though it was a little salty and bitter, was

not disgusting—but rather because I was aware of what I was doing. I forced the nausea down and rinsed my mouth immediately with coffee. I'd done it; I'd taken my first sip of morning urine. Nowadays, I am a real urine pro. For over two years now, I have drunk a glass of my urine every morning and have almost completely rid myself of hay fever, except for the rare necessity of using some eyedrops. My allergies have also diminished and my overall health has improved."

Margaret is only one of many examples. However, there are people who do not want to go so far as to drink urine but don't have to miss out on its healing effects.

Susanne Z., 28, hairdresser, reports: "When I was a child my grandmother advised me to use urine for blisters on my feet. Of course I didn't do it. I thought that would be totally disgusting. Only when I developed two giant blisters while I was hiking three years ago did I decide to try it out. I applied a few drops of urine to a cosmetic pad and kept it on my blisters over-night

(cont.)

with a Band-Aid. The next morning my blisters had opened up. With fresh Band-Aids, I was able to continue my hike without any problems. This convinced me. Today I use urine on my face (for pimples or recently when I developed a wart on my neck). The results are always astounding, the healing unbelievably fast. I think if I were faced with a chronic illness and forced to make a choice about which I would take on a daily basis, urine or medication, I would be able to drink urine, too."

The Death of Prejudice Is the Birth of the Chance to Heal

Fear about urine is conditioned and irrational. The following prejudices must be overcome:

Urine is full of germs

In the first fifteen minutes after leaving the body, urine is absolutely sterile for the producer's own body. Only after this period do the germs begin their work. However, they are not dangerous at all, and can even be beneficial for external applications. A public or badly cleaned toilet presents more hazards (fungal infections) than your own urine does.

Urine smells

After a while the uric acid in urine changes into ammonia, and only then does the urine start to smell. However, the smell will evaporate completely if the urine gets absorbed into the skin, or if, for example, it is used in the household on window glass and is thoroughly wiped off afterward.

Urine is a waste product

How can it make sense to reintroduce into the body a fluid that it just has expended considerable effort to eliminate? A short and simple explanation: Urine comprises the sum of all the experiences that the body has had (much as our individual personalities comprise the sum of our experience). Records of disturbances, infections, diseases, and allergies are stored within our urine. If we confront our immune system with this information for a second time, we stimulate the construction of a (finally) effective defense. Urine therefore teaches the immune system a lesson.

Urine develops an unpleasant odor on the skin

This is not true. It is, however, necessary for the fluid to be completely absorbed. If, for example, you make compresses, I recommend an animal fiber like wool rather than cotton, since the urine will not develop an odor in animal fibers while it will smell in cotton (as we know from cotton diapers). Urine should certainly not be used with synthetic fibers.

Urine contains viruses and bacteria

Our own urine doesn't contain any viruses or bacteria that really could harm us because those have already been filtered out by the liver. And the remaining ones are exactly the ones that the body should fight with the help of urine therapy.

Urine tastes bad

Healthy urine, especially the first evacuation in the morning, always tastes salty and bitter. This taste, however, will not be conducted through the capillaries of the tongue, but solely through the nose. If you pinch your nose while drinking, you will not taste anything.

Urine is responsible for diaper rash

This is absolute nonsense, on which the diaper industry gets rich. Urine does not harm a baby's buttocks. A sore bottom is caused solely by the infant's diet or by the diet of the nursing mother.

STILL SKEPTICAL?

Do the test!

Now it's time to take a risk and start. Forget all the thoughts that you have connected with urine since the beginning of your life. The next time you have to go to the bathroom, hold your index finger in the stream of urine. Let the liquid drip off a little and smell it. Don't be afraid: I promise you, you won't smell a thing!

Now, can you gather up even a little more courage? Then rub some of the urine on the back of your hand and wait as long as you can before you wash your hands again. You will discover that no odor will develop on your skin either. The moistened area, however, will feel softer and smoother.

Are you even more courageous? Then touch your urine-covered finger with your tongue—just very quickly. Does it taste salty? That's normal. The morning urine is especially bitter. The more fluid you take in during the day, the more "mild" the taste of urine.

The Little "Revulsion Test"

Nothing is easier said than the words "Don't make such a fuss" or "This makes you sick? Don't be ridiculous." Let's observe which situations cause you to feel disgusted (in which case, mark the "This feels very uncomfortable" column in the test on the facing page), and which situations you feel you could manage (make a mark in the "I can handle this" column). The test should make it more clear how ready you are to proceed with urine therapy. After you've finished, read the next section for an interpretation of the results of the test.

Most of your marks are in the "This feels very uncomfortable" column:

There are many things you feel revolted about. If you made around ten marks, you could be called "somewhat oversensitive." You should examine the situations that revolt you again and only progress very slowly toward drinking your urine. If you challenge yourself too much, you will lose your courage. Therefore, take it easy: Just do the finger test. If even this is asking too much from you, postpone the rubbing and tasting parts of the test to a later time. Your goal is to find a balance between overexaggerated disgust and innate sensitivity. If you find that you have a lot of difficulty with the idea of urine therapy,

Situation of disgust	This feels very uncomfortable	I can handle this
A friend belches after dinner in a restaurant.		
You see a TV ad for sanitary pads or tampons.		
A drain has to be cleaned and no tools are available. You have to use your hands.		
A friend is vomiting and needs help with cleaning up.		
Your pet has diarrhea.		
Your cat brings an almost dead mouse into the house.		
Your dog rolls in fresh cow manure.		
You find food in the household covered with mold.		
After a greasy dinner the broiler has to be cleaned.		
Your puppy is not housebroken. You have to clean up the excrement.		
Your earring disappeared in the drain and you have to empty the elbow pipe.		
You watch a man spitting on the street.		
The toilet of a bar is absolutely filthy.		
The person next to you passes gas.		

perhaps the following section, which explains how the kidneys make urine, will convince you of its potential benefits.

Most of your marks are in the "I can handle this" column:

If so, your way toward treating yourself with urine therapy will be much easier because you are able to overcome disgust to help other living beings.

Therefore, you needn't consider much longer, but rather start with the chapter "It Only Takes Effort in the Beginning."

FOR THE REAL SKEPTICS

*Our kidneys as the super sewage
system with a learning effect*

The most important prerequisite for urine therapy is this: The only people eligible for the internal use of the self-urine therapy are the ones whose bladder, kidneys, and genitals are absolutely healthy. In case of a bladder infection, a sexually transmitted disease, or the intake of certain medications (cortisone, strong pain relievers, psychopharmaceuticals, antibiotics, insulin), urine should only be used externally. Talk with your physician to see if such medications could be reduced or discontinued in favor of urine therapy.

A meal passes through your body

Regardless of whether it is solid food or a drink, until it reaches the duodenum everything goes the same way. Digestion begins with enzymes in the mouth. Then the chewed food goes down through the esophagus, a muscle pipe that forces the food mush down in the direction of the stomach. The stomach is made of muscles also, and its interior can hold about two to three liters (quarts) of fluid. From the stomach liquids pass quickly on. A soft-boiled egg remains in the stomach for about half an hour, meat for about three hours, and sardines up to nine hours. The stomach contracts rhythmically, and in its interior hydrochloric acid and pepsin break down the food.

At the stomach exit the pyloric muscles release in portions a sour, liquefied food mash into the duodenum, the 25-centimeter-long upper section of the 6-meter-long small intestine. Here the ducts of the two large digestive glands, the liver with the gallbladder and the pancreas, join into the small intestine. These digestive organs mix their juices into the food. The bile from the liver (stored in the gallbladder) emulsifies the fat, while the chyme from the pancreas contains a variety of enzymes. Under their influence, carbohydrates, fats, and proteins are broken down into simple sugars, glycerin, amino acids, and fatty acids during the long passage through the small intestine. The release of all these digestive fluids is regulated by hormones which travel through the circulatory system to relay orders to the organs.

The now nutrient-depleted food mash is pushed into the large intestine, together with one-half pound of intestinal epithelial cells, which the small intestine breaks down every day. In the large intestine billions of bacteria attack the remainder of the food and even break down the fibers of fruits and vegetables. At the same time, water is extracted from the mash in the large

How is urine actually made from food particles and drinks?
Here is a schematic and simplified diagram of the pathway.

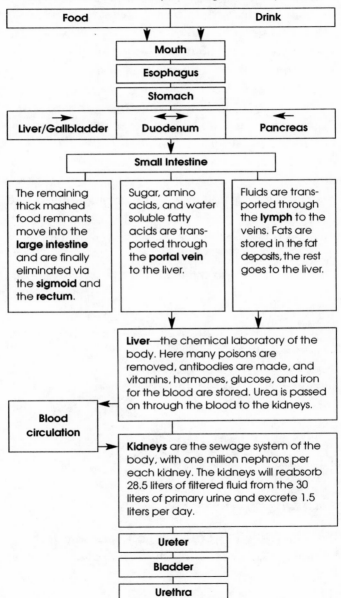

Food	Drink

Mouth

Esophagus

Stomach

Liver/Gallbladder	Duodenum	Pancreas

Small Intestine

The remaining thick mashed food remnants move into the **large intestine** and are finally eliminated via the **sigmoid** and the **rectum**.

Sugar, amino acids, and water soluble fatty acids are transported through the **portal vein** to the liver.

Fluids are transported through the **lymph** to the veins. Fats are stored in the fat deposits, the rest goes to the liver.

Liver—the chemical laboratory of the body. Here many poisons are removed, antibodies are made, and vitamins, hormones, glucose, and iron for the blood are stored. Urea is passed on through the blood to the kidneys.

Blood circulation

Kidneys are the sewage system of the body, with one million nephrons per each kidney. The kidneys will reabsorb 28.5 liters of filtered fluid from the 30 liters of primary urine and excrete 1.5 liters per day.

Ureter

Bladder

Urethra

intestine. A mushy pulp forms, consisting of brown-colored waste products, bacteria, and cell fragments: the feces, which the body expels through the anus.

The nutrients, which have been absorbed through the cells in the wall of the small intestine, are processed by the intestinal mucous membrane and passed on. Sugar and water soluble fatty and amino acids travel in the bloodstream to the portal vein and are passed on to the liver. Glycerin and insoluble fatty acids are rebuilt into fats by the intestinal cells, surrounded by proteins, and released into the tissue fluid (interstitial fluid). This enriched interstitial fluid is transported through the lymph system into the venous blood of the circulatory system. The veins transport the lymphatic fats either to the liver or to fat tissue deposit sites.

Normally, the liver weighs about five pounds, uses about one-quarter of the body's oxygen supply, and is heavily supplied with blood. It works as the chemical laboratory of the body, detoxifying the blood and storing material essential to life components such as glucose, iron, and vitamins, releasing them into the blood according to the body's demand. The liver breaks down spent proteins into urea, which is forwarded to the kidneys.

The kidneys perform clean work

Our blood flows through our liver and kidneys three hundred times a day. While the liver takes care of our chemical household, the kidneys work as our sewage system. In each of their millions of nephrons they separate blood and primary urine (glomerular filtrate), filter out the water from the filtrate (28.5 liters per day), which is reabsorbed into the body, and release 1.5 liters of urine daily into the ureter. Inside the kidneys a host of cells (nephrons), capsules, and loops are responsible for this complicated process.

Through the renal pelvis the urine flows through the ureter into the bladder. The pressure of about one liter of urine at the bladder wall will cause the bladder to empty itself into the urethra (in women a little faster than in men).

How does our body learn, anyway?

Learning is based on experience. When a small child touches something hot, he hears his mother's exclamation "hot" while simultaneously feeling the pain of a burn. His brain will memorize this experience. On the next occasion, the mother can prevent the child from touching a particular item through the simple verbal code "hot." The child has gained information from his experience and has stored it. The older a person gets, the more experiences he or she has processed and stored. The person becomes the sum of his or her experiences.

The blood and the urine in our bodies record a similar learning process. They correspond with the body's sum of experiences. Diluted parts of this experience can be found in our blood and in our urine. When these fluids are introduced to the body a second time, by employing self–transfusion therapy or self–urine therapy, the immune system will be alarmed and will step into action. This principle is called "simila similibus curentur" (to heal equal with equal). Vaccinations and homeopathy, which introduce extremely diluted pathogens into the bloodstream to stimulate immune response, are based on this principle as well. They all teach the immune system a lesson.

IT ONLY TAKES EFFORT IN THE BEGINNING

The drinking of your own urine

"Me? Drink Urine? Never!" Many patients have exclaimed these words when their therapist has suggested this form of treatment. However, the fact remains, everybody has done it before, namely in the mother's womb. The embryo has its own metabolism from the very beginning, which is connected to the mother's circulatory system. The baby gets rid of its urine just as any other human does. Therefore it also swallows its own urine constantly through the amniotic fluid. The history of humankind proves that it has not harmed anybody so far. Also, medicine has known for three thousand years that urine can be very beneficial to the small being. The Ebers Papyrus—an Egyptian book on medicine written about 1000 B.C., with a total of fifty-five recipes for urine therapy—proves this fact.

The first step

Do you have by any chance a small injury anywhere on your body, a rash, a blister, or something similar? While urinating, rub some fresh urine on it several times a day. Within a short time this spot will heal. Maybe this experience will help you gain some trust in your own juice.

The second step

Now that you have gotten over your initial disgust, can you expect even more from yourself?

Take a very clean glass. In the morning, right after getting up, try to urinate in three steps. That may sound somewhat silly, but it is meant quite seriously. The first urine to pass through the urethra cleans the passageway thoroughly. You should not collect these expelled substances. Pause briefly, position the glass, and let the urine pour in. When the glass is full, pause again. Set the glass aside and empty your bladder completely. This remaining urine does not contain many useful substances, and therefore you needn't collect it. It only would increase the amount of fluid you drink. What you have collected is the so-called morning midstream urine. This is the purest and richest urine of the day.

The third step

All right then. The urine is collected and you have fifteen minutes remaining to do something with it. Therefore, there is no need to rush. Why don't you get your favorite drink from the kitchen? No alcohol in the morning, of course, but if you expect the worst scenario (to vomit), maybe a very small and strongly spiced stomach bitter would not be inappropriate (no more than a thimbleful).

You should not push yourself now. Although you have a whole glass in front of you, a single sip that you don't spit out immediately is worth more than the entire glass that will soon end up in the toilet. Put down the glass and immediately swallow your favorite drink. Then, take a deep breath. You've done it! There, was that so terrible? I don't think so.

The fourth step

It is obvious: You have to work on increasing your daily dose until you are able to empty the whole glass. But please, don't "sweeten" your urine with a small sip of alcohol every morning. Otherwise, you are in danger of developing secondary damages, sooner or later, like dependency.

If you fail the first time

You succeeded with collecting the midstream urine, but could not go on afterward. It would be good if you could make yourself do at least the finger test, to show yourself again that urine is not disgusting. Afterward, pour the contents of the glass into the toilet. You can simply make a new attempt the next morning, and don't call yourself a "coward." Rather, be proud of how many inhibitions you have overcome already.

Make the morning drink your habit

When you reach the point where you drink your urine every morning, you are faced with an alternative:

You can do a two-week to three-month treatment course to treat a certain illness, determined by a holistic physician or by a naturopath. Or you can fight allergies or a similar chronic ailment with a continuous urine therapy (daily). In this way you provide your immune system with permanent support and achieve a lasting improvement in your general well being. If you are afraid that those around you cannot understand why you drink urine, it is better to be silent about it for now. If, however, your present complaints improve or even disappear during the treatment—and I am convinced they will—you would do our common cause a favor by talking about it. Relating your personal experiences by word of mouth would be more convincing than any book.

This was confirmed for me through the story of one of my readers:

Dale F., 54, secretary: "For years my sun allergy had ruined my vacations. My family relaxed in the sun but I had to sit in the shade under two sun umbrellas. Nevertheless, just by going swimming I broke out in fluid-filled, itching blisters. None of the sunscreen lotions helped. At a friend's I found a book on urine therapy and read that the drinking of urine would help such skin conditions. I pushed the thought aside, though, because it felt uncomfortable. During my next vacation my beach neighbor told me that her sun allergy had vanished since she started urine therapy. I started with it and today I can sit with my family next to the water."

THE QUALITY OF YOUR OWN URINE

*What your urine can reveal to you,
and how you can improve it*

The consistency and quality of urine can be influenced. People who drink less than two liters of liquid daily will notice that their urine takes on a very dark color and a stronger odor.

Unfortunately, this is often the case with older people, who can put themselves at severe medical risk by drinking too little fluid. If they don't drink enough for several days they often find their lives in danger. The entire fluid and electrolyte environment of these patients becomes completely unbalanced. Only an emergency hospital admission with IV therapy can save their lives.

Normally urine should be light yellow, and during the course of the day a total of 1.5 liters of urine should be voided. If your urine is extremely light and you have to urinate constantly, you should consult a doctor. Although the kidneys produce about 30 liters of primary urine only 1.5 liters will be passed on to the bladder. The rest is reabsorbed into the body. If the bladder suddenly excretes a lot of fluid (with the fluid intake remaining the same) it can be a symptom that indicates the kidneys are not functioning properly.

Other things to keep in mind

- ☐ Drink more fluid rather than less (and not less than two liters daily).
- ☐ Use herbs instead of salt to spice up your meals. Too much salt hinders the work of the kidneys.
- ☐ Drink seltzer water, green tea, fruit teas, or diluted juice rather than coffee (coffee dehydrates the body).
- ☐ Avoid alcohol (alcohol destabilizes the body's fluid and salt balance).

The things physicians can recognize through urine

Two things get cloudy in a sick person:
a) the urine, b) the thoughts.
—Eugen Roth

Every patient has experienced this: When a physician suspects an illness in the kidney or bladder area, the patient has to give a urine sample. Pregnancies can be detected through certain hormones found in urine as well. Physicians can also detect certain physical conditions and indicators of stress in urine, much as they can by taking a blood count. This is a centuries-old art.

In times when medicine could not gain new insights from blood, and bloodletting was the main form of treatment, urine served as the primary diagnostic tool for healers and physicians. During the Middle Ages it was taken for granted that patients would bring their morning urine to the doctor in a small flask. Here it was set aside for a while for closer examination. To arrive at a diagnosis, the urine was viewed as four layers that were supposed to correspond to four areas of the body.

Disturbances would indicate which body area was out of balance:

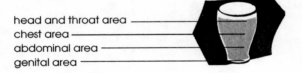

head and throat area
chest area
abdominal area
genital area

Of course, medical diagnosis isn't really that simple, but without these forerunners none of our first-class contemporary diagnostic analyses of urine would be conceivable. For example: The ancient Egyptians were aware of distinct differences in the odor of fresh urine; some of it was pungent and sour, while other samples were sweet and mild. Today it is well-known that the sweet odor is produced by glucose excreted into the urine of diabetic patients. This is the most obvious symptom of a life-threatening disease that primarily affects civilized, as opposed to primitive, peoples.

ABOUT THE RIGHT MOMENT

When is the right time to drink?

The morning midstream urine is most important for internal use because it has been in the body the longest. It is important not to collect the first portion of the urine flow, since it contains the waste that is released by the initial flushing of the urethra. The last portion also should be left for the toilet, since it contains hardly any significant ingredients. Morning midstream urine is also recommended for gargling (against gum problems and sore throats).

The fact that urine has passed through the body increases its healing effect. In this regard it acts as a stimulant to the body's immune system. The first days of urine therapy treatment can, however, lead to an initial worsening of the symptoms—a fact one should be warned about.

This means that allergies or other symptoms of disease fighting, such as fever or excessive mucus, can occur more strongly. This effect can be counteracted by diluting the morning urine (ratio 1:1) or by changing the routine (only drinking urine every other morning). If the symptoms do not improve within a week, you should talk with your therapist about them.

It is extremely important to consult a medical professional before beginning self–urine therapy, because you have to make sure that your urine is not polluted by medications or diseases. Otherwise (such as in the case of bacteria associated with a bladder infection) you could do your body more harm than good. Also, your urine's pH should be between five and seven, otherwise it can cause disturbances within the body.

Uropoty—this is the medical term for the drinking of urine—should always be done for at least fourteen days, and three months is a reasonable cycle. However, nothing can be said against drinking a glass of your urine every morning for the rest of your life. The only side effect you will experience is a mobilization of your immune system. And this can only be beneficial to your health!

Fresh urine, used externally

To tighten and tone your facial skin or to treat minor injuries, pimples, or eczema any urine can be used immediately after voiding. Fresh urine can be used for inhalation, as well. For use as nose-, ear-, or eyedrops, a fresh and, if possible, warm urine is preferred, which can be collected in a 30 ml dropper bottle (obtainable at the drugstore) at any time of the day. Compresses used for the treatment of open leg sores should be made with fresh morning urine, and applied to the wounds for approximately three hours.

To use older urine

Old urine (which has been stored for longer than fifteen minutes) generally should not be used on open wounds because it is no longer sterile. If, however, you wish to use urine to make compresses or wraps for sprains and bruises, or for a bath supplement, older urine may be used without hesitation. Old urine can be used for massages; it should not, however, be more than three to seven days old.

Sterilized urine

Naturopaths use urine in the form of injections. In this case it has to be sterilized. In the early years of urine injections (around the 1920s) phenol was added to urine to sterilize it. Today the yellow liquid is sterilized through an ozone apparatus.

Urine injection should only be peformed by a specialist, since it would be very hazardous for the patient to accidentally inject the urine into a vein or artery. In addition, only a therapist can make sure that the patient's urine is impeccable and acceptable for use in the treatment.

Old urine for the household

After two days the urea within urine begins to oxidize and an unpleasant ammonia odor appears. If you use this liquid to clean your windows, you will see how the ammonia binds with fatty deposits and wipes off without leaving streaks.

Two thousand years ago in ancient Rome, the entire laundry was cleaned with urine. So-called fullones collected the whole city's urine in big jugs, poured it into giant tubs, and stamped the laundry in it. Then the laundry was rinsed thoroughly in the river and dried in the sun. No wonder that the laundry shops were located at the edges of the city. The odor must have been horrible. By the way, the fullones had one of the best-paid professions of the times.

THE STRATEGY

*Strengthen the immune system to
build up your self-healing powers*

*Drink your own fresh and clean urine with
gratitude and joy. Every illness under which
one has suffered will be healed.*
—Indian Damar Tantra

Hippocrates (460–377 B.C.), namesake of the
Hippocratic oath, was the first in the Western
world to record and teach the practice of uropoty
(the drinking of urine). The theory of urine therapy
states: In the excreted urine all the body's experiences—physical and psychological—are collected.
Reintroducing the urine to the body forces the body's
immune system to confront the same experiences a
second time, which gives it a second incentive to deal
with the problem.

Urine functions as a nosode, a small impulse of
disease that, when introduced to the body, triggers
the healing powers of the immune system. From
homeopathy the principle of "healing like with like"
is well-known. Today's vaccinations work on the

same principle: A small impulse of an illness is introduced to the body to trigger its massive defense mechanism. In the case of immunizations one can obtain protection lasting for decades; when using urine therapy a refreshment is recommended after one year, or sometimes after just half a year.

THE PSYCHOLOGICAL EXPERIENCES OF MY PATIENTS

Suddenly I feel very close to my body

In the anal stage (between eighteen and thirty-six months of age) a child learns how to gain control over his or her body's excretions. Psychologists say that the child will use this first experience of the body's autonomy and his newfound ability against his parents. Every mother is familiar with the decision about whether to use a diaper for the long car trip: First the child says she does not want one, that she thinks she can hold it, and then with pleasure will wet her pants or terrorize everybody with constant requests for bathroom stops ("I have to go pee").

Parental praise for a filled-up potty, the pride of using the adult toilet for the first time, the first dry night without a diaper—the child will greet each of these with pleasure, provided the parents motivate their child in the right way.

> **Marion K., 32, mother of three-year-old Lisa:** "When we went out for dinner, Lisa asked us to go to the bathroom with her every three minutes. My friend and I took turns, but Lisa could not finish up. Suddenly she came back out into the dining room and yelled in her small child's voice, 'Mama I finally went.' There stood Lisa, with her overall straps hanging down. I blushed as the other guests started to laugh knowingly and the restaurant owner gave her a lollipop."

The only thing that is not allowed—and this is told to almost every child, because almost everybody tries it—is to touch or play with the potty's contents. Most parents will react with horror and say "Pee is yucky." This will limit the child's pleasure, but the parents' pride in the "potty-trained child" will compensate for the loss.

In general, this joy-filled excretion experience will end as soon as the child is able to wipe himself afterward. Then he will be asked to close the bathroom door behind himself, to wash his hands thoroughly afterward, and he realizes that nobody pays much attention to his bathroom talk anymore (how often, how much, etc.).

Boys and girls—the differences

Once children grow a little older the differences between boys and girls become more pronounced. Little boys go in to the bushes together to take a peek at how the "little distinction" looks on their friends. Competitions on who can pee the farthest are very popular. Basically, boys have a much more natural association with urination than girls do.

Little girls are lifted into a squat by their parents—the "holding over the pot" position. If girls need to go in to the bushes, they usually stay within view. The motivation here does not come from wanting to be seen but rather because they like to keep on talking. Girls also learn very early that nobody will watch them while they are urinating.

The different development of boys and girls leads to completely different public toilets, in which men continue to use urinals next to each other, while women usually use locked stalls. This strict division between "Ladies" and "Gentlemen," however, is not very common in southern European countries (where often women use stand-up toilets, as well).

Regaining joy with urine therapy

Claudia W., 54, salesclerk, told me after a few weeks of treatment: "At the beginning of the process of becoming used to urine therapy I had to deal with my excrement for the first time in half a century. I started to check the amount, color, and odor. Then I touched it, rubbed it in, and actually tried to drink it. At each step of my development I broke down inhibitions and levels of disgust and I noticed how my body—even with its excrement—became my friend. After my eczema improved through drinking urine and my sore throat got better from gargling with urine, I felt a certain pride in the substance, which I had flushed casually down the toilet before. I can describe it in another way: I have come closer to my body."

Claudia's experience is no isolated case. Urine in therapy regains the status that it held during the anal phase of a valuable product from the body, and loses its "yucky" associations.

Thomas K., 22, student, laughs nowadays about our first talks: "I really thought that you were absolutely crazy when you recommended that I should drink my urine to treat my acne. Nevertheless, three days later, I was able to carefully rub my fresh urine on my pimples. This I told you with pride and you praised me for it. At the same time you reminded me that only drinking my urine would produce lasting results against acne. Finally I overcame my inhibitions and, as promised, my acne disappeared within two months. This feeling of 'I can help myself' after all these years of being a frustrated 'pimple face' was incredible. Ever since then I have used urine therapy against all kinds of ailments. I have become my own helper!"

One of my readers found urine therapy in an unusual way and had the following experience.

Paul T., 64, retiree: "I read in your earlier book that one's own urine can be used against bedsores. For many years I have taken care of my 85-year-old mother, who has been bedridden for the last four years. Although I have help from a nurse, who comes for two hours to bathe my mother and to reposition her, she still develops open areas on her back and buttocks. Since

(cont.)

she had to use the bedpan anyway, it was easy to collect her urine. I've made compresses with it, and her open sores, which I usually need to treat for months, have indeed begun to heal very quickly. This experience has led me to trying out the therapy on myself. As I often felt very burdened with my nursing care, I frequently felt sick myself, and I hoped that I could strengthen my immune system. And what a surprise: Today I feel stronger, more efficient, and healthy. The ability to heal myself has always been within me. An indescribable feeling."

COCKTAIL HOUR

*Experiences with urine combined
with other healing remedies*

The healing effects of urine can be increased through
the addition of other natural remedies. Here are some
recipes from my practice and from my patients.

Arnica helps against the tendency to bruise, against
   hematoma below the skin, and against fistula.

Bach flowers work especially well in psychosomatic
   diseases. They give an additional impulse to the psyche to activate the immune system for self-healing.

Chamomile extract (tincture) supports the healing
   effect of fresh urine against external infections and
   moderates any discomfort associated with nasal
   urine therapy (nosedrops).

Cimicifuga supports urine therapy in women's diseases and in hormone stimulation (during the
   menopause years).

Dandelion stimulates gallbladder function for digestive problems and gallstones.

Digitalis in homeopathic form plus a basic urine therapy serve together to strengthen the heart.

Echinacea strengthens the body's immune system.

Fango compresses are a wonderful support for all diseases that have to do with the skeletal system. I also recommend physical therapy for my patients.

Ginkgo (the sap of the tree), either in homeopathic form or pure, can help with circulation disorders.

Hamamelis is a good remedy for varicose veins and hemorrhoids and as a complement to urine therapy.

Ignatia (from the Ignatius bean) relieves cramps, migraines, and other diseases.

Juniper stimulates the kidneys and has a diuretic effect, effective against tissue edema and kidney stones.

Mercury in a homeopathic form (extremely diluted) works as an antiseptic and antibacterial. It is especially effective in combatting infections in the throat.

Okoubaka (West African tree) is a very good additional therapy for stomach problems and poisoning of the digestive tract.

Pulsatilla is the remedy that I give to adolescent girls and women for menstrual problems.

Rosemary has a stimulating effect against exhaustion and fatigue.

Salt from the Dead Sea supports urine therapy as a bathing salt or as a compress in cases of skin diseases like psoriasis and neurodermatitis.

Sodium chloride (table salt) can be used as an addition to urine for gargling. It is very friendly to skin and mucous membranes.

Spleen preparations are good remedies to support urine therapy for problems during menopause.

St. John's wort is very helpful against depression, similar to basic urine therapy, and can be used in addition (as a tea or in capsules). It is especially effective for women (for men see *zinc valerianicum*).

Thymus (a fresh cell preparation from the thymus gland) as a lozenge or an injection helps against immune deficiency and recurrent infections and has a rejuvenating effect.

Urtica (stinging nettle) can be taken against gout and rheumatism in conjunction with urine massages.

Viscum album (mistletoe) is effective against hypertension (high blood pressure) and supports circulation.

Yohimbe (tree bark) is an excellent remedy for increasing potency (prescribed as a series of injections in addition to fasting with urine).

Zinc valerianicum calms the nerves and stabilizes the nervous system especially for men (for women see *St. John's wort*).

A QUICK COURSE IN TREATING YOURSELF

~~*❧*~~   ~~*❧*~~

*Urine applications as inhalations,
compresses, and drinks*

External Application

The external application of urine can be seen as a kind of first aid. Small injuries, sprains, burns, etc., are treated directly with fresh urine. When one lives on a farm, this can be done not only with one's own urine but also with the cattle's urine. However, urine from cattle should not be applied to open wounds.

Small areas of application like pimples, warts, age spots, eczema, or ugly scars can be wetted several times a day. If you don't want to have the urine on your fingers, you can use a cotton swab.

Midstream morning urine is very effective and odorless for rubbing into the skin. Acne, dry or oily facial skin, the first wrinkles—all of them can be cleared and eliminated by rubbing the first urine onto the face in the morning. For the rest of the body you may also use older urine, which has already developed an ammonia odor. The odor will disappear after the urine has been absorbed into the skin. Applications onto areas of pain should be made twice daily; after fourteen days you may take a break for one week.

Wraps, Dressings, and Compresses

Wraps, dressings, and compresses are also external applications. One rule is extremely important: Never use urine on synthetics. Linings should always be made out of natural fiber materials. If wool can be tolerated against the skin, it is the best for preventing odor, but linen or cotton make acceptable linings as well. For open wounds only fresh and therefore sterile urine can be used. For sprains, sciatica, or similar conditions collected urine may be used, and it may be warmed up prior to use. A fresh cloth is dipped into the urine to make the compress. The following needs to be noted, though: If the area is red, hot, or inflamed (without open festering sores or furuncles) the wraps must be cold and should be exchanged after they have warmed up. This can be done with only two wraps, with one always chilling while the other is in use.

Massage

Although the cheapest and best remedy, urine is rarely recommended for massage. But a urine massage provides a great alternative whether you massage your partner, your children, or yourself. Nothing regenerates weakened skin (due to a damaged pH balance) faster or better. If the problem is tension in the neck, a sore muscle, tennis elbow, or cramps, nothing is more effective than the residue-free massage of urine into the skin. The urine should be between three and six days old (therefore, keep collecting it). Since urine has a blood thinning effect, it will generate a very pleasant warming circulation. Anybody who has aesthetic difficulties with a urine massage can take a shower afterward (but please, no soap or bath oil).

Baths

Urine baths are taken by adding about one liter of urine (collected within one week) to a bathtub full of water. Possible problems with the odor can be eliminated by taking a shower afterward (no soap, no shower gel). Sitz baths or small eye baths (see *Sty*) are also possible.

Drinking

This is the internal application, the so-called uropoty. Most often the basic urine therapy is recommended. This consists of drinking one glass of midstream urine every morning for a period of six weeks followed by a one-week break. If the complaints have subsided, the therapy may be ended. If the symptoms reappear, take two sips of urine in the morning for a short period. A person who drinks his or her urine daily provides great support for the immune system. The daily routine will also diminish the disgust. "Professional" urine drinkers report that they don't rinse their mouths afterward and have never felt better.

When urine is used internally an initial worsening of the symptoms can be expected. Allergies or similar complaints will appear more severely for a short time period. If the symptoms don't improve quickly, drinking urine every other day is recommended.

Fasting with Urine

Urine fasting is the most intense treatment because additional healing incentives are given to the detoxifying body through the urine. In addition, the use of laxatives can be avoided if each excreted urine is given back to the body. A urine fasting course should last a minimum of five days and a maximum of three weeks and should be supervised by a therapist (physician or naturopath). The patient has to drink two to three liters of water in addition to the urine and take a specific combination of vitamins and minerals, which will be recommended by the therapist. Due to the increase of lactic acid in the muscles lots of exercise is important. The ending of the fast is also very important: On the first day after the fast only a steamed apple and a thin potato, rice, or vegetable broth should be eaten. On the second day rusk or crisp bread is added to each meal. Unpeeled boiled potatoes with fat-free cottage cheese is also a reasonable meal for the next days. Fat and meat, as well as alcohol, should be avoided. And choose a special time for this fast, which should be done once a year, like the week before Easter or five days before your birthday.

Gargling

In the time before penicillin children with diphtheria had to gargle with morning urine. In many cases this "grandmother recipe" prevented the swelling and closing of the larynx and saved the children's lives. For tonsillitis, sore throats, and mouth ulcers gargling with urine is still an adequate treatment. It is important that the fluid be kept in the mouth or throat for as long as possible. This makes it more effective.

If the morning midstream urine is too salty or bitter, it can be diluted with water in a 1:1 ratio. A little sunflower oil or a few drops of chamomile tincture can make this procedure easier and help reduce the infection. The recommended course for gargling in the mouth is four days a week with a one week intermission and so on.

Enema

Especially for toddlers and infants, enemas offer a good way to administer urine therapy. The child is placed on its side, both knees are pulled toward the chest, and with a bulb syringe (babies 1 to 3 ml, older children about 5 ml) the urine is injected into the rectum. For this procedure one can also use a syringe (without the needle, of course).

Adults should use 10 to 40 ml as an "indwelling enema" (which means that the fluid will be absorbed completely by the intestinal wall). A urine enema should consist of one part urine and one part lukewarm chamomile tea or water. An irrigator should be used in an adult to administer the enema and somebody should help with the procedure.

It is important that the mixture be retained in the colon as long as possible. The best way is to position the patient on the back and to gently massage the abdomen in a clockwise direction. The strong urge to evacuate will only increase the detoxification.

Quantities for the Intestinal Flush	
(evacuated enema)	
Babies	5 ml
Children	up to 1000 ml
Adults	1 to 2 liters

Injection

In Germany urine injections have been administered since 1920. This technique, however, can be administered only by an experienced therapist (physician or naturopath). In the first decades, phenol was added to the urine injections. Today the urine is sterilized with an ozone treatment.

Therefore, this information is for the therapist: The injection is done with a 20-gauge needle subcutaneously (directly under the skin). The quantity can be increased from 0.5 ml to a maximum of 5 ml. Injections should be given only every two days. Injection therapy has proven beneficial for menopausal problems, allergies, and asthma. Injections also can be given directly into the muscle, which speeds up the distribution of the urine. Under no circumstances should urine be injected into veins or arteries.

Drops and Homeopathy

Nose, ears, and eyes can be treated with a dropper bottle (30 cc pipette, available through drugstores). For nosedrops one should use fresh, warm urine, most preferably the morning urine. Even if applications will be made frequently throughout the day, one should always use the freshest urine that has not been previously collected. For the treatment of all mucous membranes it is important to use sterile urine.

The same is true for eardrops, which are always used undiluted. One should plug the ear with an oil-soaked cotton ball to ensure that the urine remains in the ear for an effective treatment period.

The first urine contains too much salt to be used as eyedrops; any other urine may be used. However it should be diluted in a ratio of one part urine to five parts distilled water or chamomile tea.

Homeopathy is the only treatment area in which urine that is infected through a bladder or kidney infection may be used. This might even lead to recovery from these diseases. The reason for this surprising advice is based on the strong dilution of the infected urine. Homeopathy (with its principle of healing equal with equal) assumes that the impulse of the immune system to fight an intruder is all the stronger the smaller the initial impulse is. The dilution is made in the following way. Take several 20 cc bottles (with screw-on lids) and fill the first one with 1 cc of urine (morning midstream urine). Add 9 cc of water and shake vigorously. Now, take 1 cc of this solution, pour it into the second bottle, and add another 9 cc of water. Altogether, this procedure must be repeated six times. Of this final dilution, children should drink five drops three times a day and adults ten drops.

Inhalation

For respiratory illnesses from colds to bronchitis, urine inhalations are extremely helpful. Add one teaspoon of your urine to a ten-quart bowl of hot water. Place your head over the bowl and cover it with a big towel. Inhale until the hot steam no longer rises. (It is permissable to take an outside breath now and then.) Of course you also can buy an inhalator from the drugstore.

TREATMENT RESULTS
AND APPLICATIONS

For Ailments from Head to Toe

Head/Throat

Canker sores

Anybody who suffers from these painful sores inside the mouth will be willing to try out the unusual. The sufferer should gargle with urine twice a day. If the morning urine tastes too bitter or salty, it can be mixed with chamomile tea or clear water (1:1). Between garglings one can dip a Q-tip into urine and rub it on the infected areas. It is important to push the urine through the teeth and swish it inside the mouth. The longer it is gargled the more effective this treatment will be.

> **George B., 53, offset printmaker,** suffered for years from mouth sores. Only after using urine therapy was he able to manage his problem. Altogether, he had to undergo the procedure for six months before the last sore disappeared. Amazingly, George has been without any symptoms for two years now.

Cataracts/Glaucoma

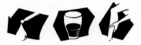

In the progressed stage of this illness only an operation can really help. However, at the first sign of cataracts in the eyes one can achieve some results with urine therapy. The following combination is recommended: Eye irrigation in the evenings (see *Sty*), eyedrops (see *Conjunctivitis*) during the day for six weeks. This is followed by a six-week course of urine drinking and then again eyedrops and baths. It is worth a try, especially if it can postpone the operation for a few years.

The same therapy is used for glaucoma as for cataracts. If the glaucoma is associated with bad headaches, the temples and the areas behind the ears should be massaged with urine after each urination. Be sure to have your ocular pressure monitored regularly, in any case, since unchecked glaucoma can cause blindness.

Frank D., 58, construction worker, came to me after his physician had diagnosed him with glaucoma. He admitted: "I've already heard from my mother that the surgery is not so bad, but to be honest, I don't want to go under the knife. I'm afraid of it." He stuck with my recommended therapy and for three years his ocular pressure has not deteriorated.

Conjunctivitis (pinkeye)

> **Christina Z., 12, student,** has suffered since the age of four from chronic conjunctivitis. Although the condition was not very painful, the stuck eyelids in the morning and the constant red eyes were a real nuisance. Christina was an expert in the use of eyedrops, but after trying many different preparations, she had found none effective. Her mother introduced her to me and I suggested urine therapy. Finally, Christina's symptoms have cleared up.

The treatment for eyes is the following: In a 30 cc dropper bottle from the drugstore mix a solution of ⅘ distilled water and ⅕ absolutely fresh urine. Put two drops in each eye. This will burn. If the feeling doesn't subside after five minutes, rinse with water.

Ear pain/Middle ear infection (otitis media)

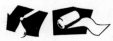

Since the hearing duct, nose, throat, and sinuses are connected with each other, extreme earaches can be fought with eardrops as well as nosedrops. With a

30 cc dropper bottle (obtainable at the drugstore), instill fresh urine in all four orifices every two hours. The ear should be plugged with a cotton ball soaked in oil. The oil prevents the cotton from absorbing the urine. To prevent odor, the ear should be rinsed carefully with warm water once a day.

Hannah T., 9, student, came with her mother to my office. She suffered from a bad ear infection, had a slight fever, and had no appetite. I advised her mother to treat Hannah's ears with fresh urine eardrops and to start six weeks of basic urine therapy as well to support the immune system, which was already fighting the infection with the fever. After beginning the eardrops Hannah was pain-free within two days and completely improved within a week.

Eczema of the ear canal

A rash inside the outer ear duct also responds well to urine therapy. For this purpose once again fill a dropper bottle with fresh urine. Every morning and evening insert three fresh drops into the ear canal, and normally the rash will be gone within days.

Hair loss

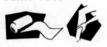

> **Thorsten H., 19, baker,** visited my office with a very special problem: "In the last half year I have lost a frightening amount of hair. You can probably already see my receding hairline. I don't want to become as bald as my father was when he was my age." My advice: urine therapy. Since then Thorsten's hair loss has indeed been stopped.

Collect urine for three days in a closed bottle. It will oxidize and won't smell very good. Spread this solution through the hair. The foaming of the urine cleans the hair thoroughly. Afterward, rinse for a while but do not apply any other remedies (conditioners or rinses) to the hair. Now massage the scalp with fresh urine, put on a shower cap, and go to bed (it has to stay on for at least six hours). Underneath the shower cap—and I don't want to conceal this—a strong ammonia odor will form. In the morning wash your hair as usual.

Headache

The drinking of urine helps for internal reasons. In the case of tension headaches the therapist may inject urine into the painful area (as described for cervical spine complaints). In milder cases massaging the neck, temples, and behind the ears with cool urine might be sufficient help.

Ronald W., 26, computer specialist, has suffered since childhood from headaches for which neither a neurologist nor an internist nor an ophthalmologist could find the cause. He writes: "A girlfriend recommended her naturopath to me and I decided to try one more time. Although the fundamental urine therapy felt very awkward (Who really likes to drink urine?) after ten days the attacks started to subside. I held out for six weeks longer and repeat the therapy once every half year. Now, when my headaches come back, they are less intense and I can cure them with a massage. The pharmaceutical industry has lost a good customer in me."

Hearing

I want to be sure not to create any misunderstandings: Real hearing loss cannot be countered with urine. However, in cases of minor, primary (age-related) hearing weaknesses, minor reduction in hearing, or tinnitus a trial with urine eardrops should be undertaken. For this we need the dropper bottle from the drugstore again (30 cc). We fill it up with fresh, warm urine and instill several drops into each ear (for best results the patient should lie on his or her side). Afterward, plug the ear with an oil-soaked cotton ball and leave it in place overnight. In the morning you must clean your ears thoroughly, since the urine will generate an odor. If you experience no positive results within six weeks, you should consult a physician or naturopath again, since the problem might be more severe than anticipated.

> **Ken K., 59, doorman,** did not notice anything until a colleague approached him. "It was around ten o'clock at night, as I was sitting in the porter's office, when an accountant asked me whether I had problems with my ears. He referred to the loud volume of my TV. This was very embarrassing for me. In your first book on urine therapy I found the advice about eardrops. And really, after four weeks my symptoms were gone. I thanked the colleague from the accounting office again and I told him why I can hear better now."

Hoarseness

The same applies here as for sore throats: The earlier you start the urine therapy the greater the chances for success. If you start to gargle with a 1:1 urine to water mixture when you feel the first scratch in your throat you can eradicate the symptoms in record time.

> **Olivia T., 38, who sings in her free time in the church choir,** went to her physician before she decided to see me as a naturopath. "My doctor could not figure out why I get sore throats frequently before concerts. I am absolutely desperate, since I really love to be part of these concerts." I recommended urine therapy and also advised her to drink her urine for at least fourteen days prior to the concerts, since I suspected that the symptoms could result from stage fright. Since starting urine therapy, Olivia has been on concert tours with her choir and has had no further problems with her throat. If it starts scratching, she immediately starts gargling.

Migraine

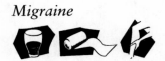

Conventional medicine has had only mixed success in treating migraine headaches. There are several medications against migraines on the market, but they don't work for all sufferers and repeated use tends to diminish their effectiveness. The causes of migraines are not fully understood but we do know that women are more frequently affected than men; the pain usually occurs unilaterally; and attacks usually do not last longer than twenty-four hours. Other symptoms associated with migraine are nausea, dizziness, vomiting, and blurry vision or partial loss of the vision field. Neural therapy and acupuncture have shown good results in the treatment of this chronic illness. It is also worthwhile to try the basic urine therapy (drinking the midstream urine every morning for six weeks). In addition, one can also massage the forehead, the area behind the ears, and the neck with urine. If the attacks don't reappear within three months the therapy may be stopped. For light attacks a massage or a washcloth soaked in urine and placed on the neck or forehead are helpful.

Nasal congestion

Nosedrops made from freshly collected urine (use a pipette from the drugstore) are very effective, but not very pleasant to use. If the burning sensation is too unpleasant, chamomile tea or water with chamomile tincture can be added (1:1). Within twenty-four hours the cold symptoms will be improved. As soon as the nose is completely back to normal the therapy may be terminated.

Nasal drip (allergies)

People with allergies are especially familiar with this symptom. Most often a cold is not the reason for this annoying runny nose; rather, it is caused by an allergic reaction (often accompanied by tearing eyes, sneezing, and swollen mucous membranes). With every urination some of the fresh urine should be collected in a dropper bottle. A few drops should be squirted into each nostril at once. This will burn, but it will help within days. The treatment should last until the sniffles are gone.

Annette J., 42, bookseller, was rather desperate when she came into my office. With all her sneezing she could hardly tend to her customers. After conducting an allergy test, it was determined that she had an allergic reaction to house dust (which of course is rather widespread in a bookstore). As a quick solution I recommended urine nasal drops. In addition I asked the patient to get accustomed to the drinking of urine, so that her body would lose its hypersensitivity. After four days her sniffles were already gone, and after she drank urine for three months her allergy had disappeared.

Neck pain and cervical spine complaints

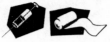

It is difficult to combine all these symptoms under one topic, since they stretch from tension in the neck to tennis elbow to headaches that are caused by tension in the neck. As a first-aid step use a washcloth that has been soaked in urine and place it on the neck for half an hour (draped by a warm towel). If you leave the cloth on for the whole night, it makes more sense to use a 1:1 urine to warm water mixture. This will not smell as bad the next morning. A trained practitioner might administer urine injections to the affected area. Since urine injected under the skin feels very painful, the therapist would use procaine in addition.

Periodontal problems

As with every condition that has to do with mucous membranes, fresh (sterile) urine should be used. The receding gum line can be treated with urine therapy only if the problems are really new. Already existing damage cannot be reversed (such as gum pockets). The best treatment is to gargle with urine every morning accompanied by the basic urine therapy, which strengthens the immune system. The liquid should be squeezed and sucked through the teeth several times.

Andrea L., 37, shipping agent, wrote to me about her experience with the first urine therapy book: "When my dentist informed me that I showed the first signs of periodontal infection I became quite frightened because I had seen how my mother lost all her teeth at the age of 40 due to the same disease. I was afraid the same thing would happen to me. Therefore I tried your recipe and I continue using it. My dentist praised me because my gums look healthier now. When I told him what I did he was very interested, since I was not the first patient of his who had tried your advice."

Scalp (dandruff, Candida albicans *infection)*

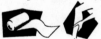

An itching scalp and dandruff are a real anguish that cannot be eliminated even with the most expensive shampoo (this applies for dry as well as oily hair). Urine should be collected for an entire day and applied to the scalp in the evening just before bed (massage it in deeply). The hair should then be covered with a shower cap and in addition, if desired, you may wrap a towel around it to keep it warm. The urine works throughout the night by stimulating the circulation and thereby regenerates the scalp from the inside. In the morning rinse vigorously with warm water (without shampoo).

Ellen K., 69, writes: "My hair was always perfect. Four years ago I suddenly developed dandruff. I tried every shampoo on the market but most of them just dried my hair out, turning it to straw. Then I read your advice on urine therapy and I remembered a remedy that my mother had recommended to me, to wrap the head with urine overnight. Now my dandruff is gone. If I find some occasionally, I make a new wrap, which takes care of it within one night."

Sinus cavity

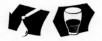

The general rule is: Whenever urine penetrates into the mucous membranes it does not feel very good, since the salt works very harshly during the healing. Therefore, anybody who is very sensitive to pain should use a 1:1 water to urine mixture. In the case of a sinus infection the following therapy is recommended: At least once a day fill a 30 cc dropper bottle with fresh urine, still warm (or the mixture of urine and warm water), lie down, and instill several drops into each nostril.

Even more effective is a nasal rinse: Buy an irrigation syringe in the drugstore and fill it with a 1:1 solution of one part warm water with a teaspoon of sea salt dissolved in it to one part fresh urine. With your head over the sink, put the pipe end into your nostril and raise the irrigator, so that the saltwater-urine mixture can run into the nose. It rinses the sinus cavities, disinfects, and comes out the other nostril. Use half of the solution for one nostril and repeat with the remainder for the other nostril. Twenty-five drops of chamomile tincture or a teaspoon of sunflower oil will make the treatment more pleasant. For chronic sinusitis an additional six-week-long basic therapy with daily drinking of urine is recommended.

Sarah H., 26, radio announcer, came to my office one day: "My boss sent me to see you. He complains that I speak with too much of a nasal tone. For years I have been treated for chronic sinus infections. Despite high dosages of antibiotics my symptoms always reoccur." The patient was not afraid of urine therapy. Therefore it was possible to start with the first nasal irrigation right in my office. She took the irrigation device home and in addition started to drink her urine every day for six weeks. Her nasal voice subsided after two weeks, and for half a year Sarah has been completely free of symptoms.

Sore throat

Almost sensational results can be obtained for throat conditions with urine therapy. The earlier one starts the treatment the faster the problem can be brought under control. For best results you should start gargling when you feel the very first scratch in your throat. Basically, any fresh urine can be used throughout the day. The liquid should be held in the throat for at least one minute. Rinse with water afterward. It is astonishing to see how urine not only dissolves the abscesses, but also activates the self-healing mechanism of the body, thereby preventing the occurrence of the next infection.

Stroke

Urine therapy cannot help much after the damage has been done. However, through drinking the morning urine, employing urine enemas, and even with urine massages a stroke might be prevented. Urine thins the blood and inhibits the formation of blood clots that can plug the arteries. In conjunction with a proper diet, a balanced workout, and continued medical screening of blood parameters, the danger can be warded off.

Sty

> **Petra M., 27, hairdresser,** had suffered for
> years from frequently recurrent stys on her
> eye. Finally, I gave her the saving advice:
> urine therapy. After only three days of
> treatment the sty had cleared up. So far,
> Petra has not needed another treatment.

Fill a small eye basin (available in drugstores) with
⅘ distilled water and ⅕ fresh urine (not the very
strong morning urine, but any consecutive one). The
affected eye is bathed in it for several minutes. The eye
can even be opened but it is not required since the
urine will reach the eyelid through the eyelashes.

Thrush (Candida albicans)

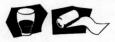

Toddlers and infants are especially affected by this
disease, which is marked by white patches in the oral
cavity. Therefore the best treatment method, namely
gargling with urine, is rather difficult to accomplish.
For infants mothers can use a knotted gauze pad,
which the baby can suck on. Feelings of disgust have

not yet developed very far in these little people. For toddlers it is easier to wipe the mouth with fresh urine than to try to get the child to gargle. Within a few days the symptoms will be gone.

Trigemminal neuralgia (Bell's palsy)

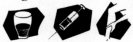

The trigemminal nerve is one of the main central nerves and has three branches (when looked at from the side). The upper one starts at the tip of the nose and runs over the eyes to the brain. The second branch reaches from the edge of the mouth to the upper brain. And the third one goes from the chin toward the ears and into the brain. There are different kinds of trigemminal neuralgia with entirely different clinical pictures.

> **Patricia B., 55, dental technician,** was exhausted when she came to my office. She complained of very strong left-sided headaches, suffered with nervous facial spasms on the left side, and had tearing eyes and a reddened face. When I palpated specific nerve points I triggered another pain attack. This is a typical picture especially in women over fifty. I advised urine injections. This treatment method, in which urine is injected

under the skin, is not very pleasant. It burns badly. The injected urine has to be massaged in. Urine eardrops and rubbing urine behind the ears, on the forehead, and on the neck also proved beneficial. Patricia soon felt better, but to be on the safe side she used the basic urine therapy in addition.

Vertigo

There are many serious reasons for vertigo. Therefore, the symptoms must be examined carefully first. If the cause, however, proves to be a mild circulatory problem or something of that nature, the following urine therapy is good advice: Every morning and every night fresh urine should be rubbed on the neck and into the hairline. In addition, every time you wash your hair before shampooing massage some urine into the scalp and let it work for at least an hour.

Wrinkles

Nobody can escape the aging process. However, millions of women succumb to the promises of the cosmetic industry, believing that the symptoms of aging can be at least temporarily postponed. They don't realize that their own bodies produce the cheapest and best antiwrinkle cream of all time. In the morning and evening the hands should be held briefly in urine and the liquid spread over face, neck, and chest. Massage it in thoroughly so that no odor can develop. Your partner will never know how you achieved such smooth, tight skin.

Chest

Asthma

More and more children and adults suffer from sudden onset of breathing problems. The reasons for this condition can vary greatly. Often, they are of a psychosomatic nature. Psychological causes for asthma often imply a compulsive need for cleanliness. Sometimes allergies or heart disease can also trigger asthma.

> **Harris P., 19, high school honor student,** had suffered from asthma since his early childhood. During the first interview in my office it became clear that Harris would react almost hysterically to the first signs

of dirt. He became even more upset when I suggested a basic urine therapy. Four more sessions went by before Harris finally promised: "Tomorrow I'll do it." I knew him well enough to know that he would keep his promise. He completed the six weeks and has not had an attack since. My experience tells me that breaking through his feelings of fear and disgust might have helped him more than the urine itself.

Bronchitis/Cough

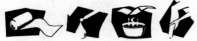

Urine chest compresses should always be cold (change them when they warm up). Fresh urine is not required; the older fluid has an even better penetrating effect, increases the circulation, and redirects waste products from the tissue. The urine can also be massaged directly into the skin or used for inhalation (one teaspoon of urine added to the water of the inhalator). Nosedrops can also help.

Cold

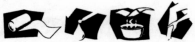

See *Bronchitis/Cough* or *Nasal congestion*.

Cyanosis

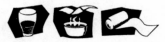

This blue and red discoloration of skin and mucous membranes is mostly due to a lack of oxygen supply to the affected areas and should be thoroughly examined. In milder cases, with the lips turning blue in conjunction with difficulties breathing (be aware that this also can indicate a cardiac problem), urine inhalation can help. A basic urine therapy can also improve the circulation. In addition, the affected body parts can be treated with compresses.

Emphysema (decreased air exchange within the lung)

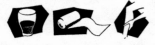

In the acute phase of emphysema urine therapy will not be enough support. However, with the very first appearance of hourglass fingernails, drumstick fingers, difficulty breathing with coughing fits, or cyanotic lips, urine compresses on the chest can feel soothing. In addition, a basic urine therapy is recommended and daily rubdowns with urine at night can be very beneficial.

> **Keith S., 24, student,** had pulmonary edema due to asthma and constantly suffered from shortness of breath. He could not participate in sports activities anymore, which was especially bad, since he studied physical education. I ordered an all-around urine therapy and he was able to breathe better within days.

Heart attack

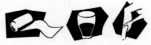

Not much can be achieved with urine therapy after a heart attack. But a heart attack might be prevented through the drinking of urine in the morning, by employing urine enemas, and even by administering urine massages or urine compresses on the chest. Urine thins the blood and prevents the formation of blood clots that can plug arteries. In conjunction with other important factors like the right diet, a balanced exercise program, and constant medical monitoring of blood and cardiac markers, the danger of getting a heart attack can be greatly reduced.

Carsten P., 48, manager, had always had a very muscular body. Since he was a young man he had gone to the health club or jogged after work. However, at the time of his first visit he had not exercised for quite a while, and his muscles were decreasing while his beer belly was increasing. He also smelled of cigarette smoke. Mr. P. told me the reason for his office visit: "My doctor found elevated cholesterol levels in my blood. He cautioned me about a heart attack and forbade me to drink alcohol. I really try. After all, I still have little children. But I would feel less afraid if I were doing more." It is relatively easy to suggest urine therapy to such a motivated patient. In his case it will have two very beneficial effects: First, his blood will thin out more and second, the drinking of the morning urine will have a positive effect on the patient's feelings of fear. Of course, I agreed with his doctor about the alcohol prohibition and recommended a careful exercise plan (five minutes of gymnastics in the morning in front of an open window, gradually increasing, but under no circumstances jogging in place). A fat-free diet was also necessary for Carsten. At his last checkup he had lost 15 pounds and showed acceptable blood results.

Arms/Hands

Arthritis

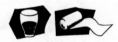

Inflammation in the joints is very painful. When treating these cases with urine it is important that the compresses be somewhat cold rather than warm. About every fifteen minutes the compress should be changed. It is also very beneficial to drink two sips of urine with each urination. After six weeks the therapy should pause for one week. If the compresses cause the skin to redden they should only be applied every other day.

Arthrosis

> **Luise W., 79, retired,** suffered from degen-
> erative joints and could only walk with a
> cane. She hardly went outside anymore and
> experienced a lot of pain. Then a therapist
> tried urine in conjunction with the intake of
> gelatin (every morning) and eight injections
> of a fresh cell preparation. In addition, urine
> was injected underneath the skin above the
> painful joints. This was a rather unpleasant
> form of treatment, but it was successful.
> Luise can now climb stairs again. The ther-
> apy must be repeated every two years.

Another form of treatment is the use of urine compresses, which should be applied daily and then covered with a soft towel (this warms the affected area
and protects the bedsheets). They must stay on for at
least half an hour. After the tenth treatment, a one
week break is indicated, then the whole course
should start again until the pain has markedly subsided. In the morning and afternoon one should
drink one or two sips of urine, which is also beneficial. Please note that degenerative joint changes cannot be reversed, but the pains they cause can be
reduced.

Hands (chapped, rough)

If you always have bought the most expensive hand cream yet still suffer from rough and chapped hands, you should try the cheapest recipe in the world. Use your last urine before you go to bed and rub your hands with it until the fluid is completely gone. Once the urine is completely absorbed by the skin your hands will not smell, and you will notice that they are in much better condition after three days. Small cracks can heal extremely well in this way.

Nails

> **Sylvia B., 19, hairdresser,** was at wit's end when she finally came to me: "I manicure my customers' nails but my own break constantly, which cannot be the best advertisement for our manicure." She followed my advice, bathing her fingers in urine every morning and evening, and after three weeks she had lovely long fingernails again.

Fill a small bowl with urine and move the hands (one after the other) back and forth in the bath. Afterward, do not wash the hands but dry them thoroughly. In this way, odor will not develop.

Warts

Anybody who has had a dermatologist freeze warts on their hands might be ready to try out a less painful procedure: After each urination apply fresh urine to the wart. Within a week the problem should be completely gone.

Cynthia A., 12, student, wrote to me: "I had warts for a long time and really felt disgusted by them. Once the dermatologist froze them. First I didn't feel anything, but then it started to hurt. My mother read to me from her book on urine therapy and told me that I should try it. After only five days the whole nuisance was over! If I look at my hands today and find something that looks like a wart I immediately start with the right treatment—and get rid of it."

Abdomen/Back

Abdominal pain

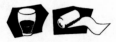

The most frequent reasons for abdominal pain are psychosomatic in nature. Stress, fear, and anger trigger an overproduction of stomach acid. This causes cramping in the area of the stomach's exit, irritation of the mucous membrane, inflammation (gastritis), and finally possible stomach ulcers. These will heal up but each scar in the mucosa of the stomach can be the cause for a new colic.

Ulrich B., 42, entrepreneur, wrote: "For years I suffered with stomach problems. Then, I read your first book and started to drink my urine. First I drank a sip whenever I urinated, then I changed to drinking one glass of midstream urine every morning. I treated acute pain with warm urine compresses. In addition I changed my diet a little, stopped drinking coffee, and I avoid spicy or salty meals. I have been free of symptoms for half a year. To be on the safe side, I continue with my morning drink."

Bloating/Flatulence (organ dysfunctions, Candida albicans)

The causes for frequent or even chronic flatulence should be examined by a doctor or naturopath. Malfunctions of the liver, gallbladder, or pancreas can cause this complaint. In acute cases (after eating gas-forming food) drinking fresh urine just once could help. Small enemas also help to break down the unpleasant flatulence.

Greg F., 28, mechanic, came to me. The reason: "My friends make fun of my 'beer belly.' I haven't even gained weight but for the last few days I have had a lot of gas. Throughout the day—especially after every meal—I feel as though I'm filled up with air." To find the cause for his complaint I first asked him for a stool sample. And indeed: Yeast was found in the intestine *(Candida albicans)*. The patient started with an intestinal regeneration course, which will reconstitute the intestinal flora. The therapy consists of the antifungal medicine Nystatin and urine enemas (small ones, so the intestine can absorb them) as well as a special antifungal diet, with total abstinence from sugar and white flour for at least two weeks.

Constipation

> **Iris J., 52, secretary,** had suffered for twenty
> years from constipation and had tried
> almost every over-the-counter laxative
> (leading to addiction). Without medication
> her bowels would not move. I was not very
> surprised since the peristaltic (smooth
> muscle movement) of the intestine gets
> used to the external motivation of medica-
> tions and loses its own natural motivation.
> This state of affairs had led to the occur-
> rence of a bloated abdomen in Iris's case.
> Since the danger of electrolyte loss through
> laxatives also existed (in which case many
> important minerals are lost for the metab-
> olism), I advised her to take the basic urine
> therapy and to perform abdominal exer-
> cises in the morning. Within a short time
> her daily bowel movement had returned to
> normal—completely without pills.

The patient drank her morning midstream urine
every day and in addition routinely did two minutes
of gymnastics before breakfast. After six weeks she
was able to terminate the therapy. In the case of miss-
ing a bowel movement for a day, she drinks two sips
of her urine and everything is back in order.

Diarrhea

First rule: fasting and lots of fluids. Nothing cures diarrhea as well as the total renunciation of food. Small urine enemas (5 cc twice daily) can also be recommended.

Diverticuli

Just as these pouches begin to form in the intestine the use of a nonretaining enema could be beneficial. For this enema one to two liters of fluid is needed (one part chamomile tea, one part urine). It is also necessary to have a therapist who can ensure the calm process of the treatment. The fluid should be retained within the colon for as long as possible. The patient should lie on his or her back while the therapist massages the abdomen counterclockwise. The urine stimulates the excretion reflex and extracts poison from the intestine. All the abdominal organs are stimulated and the intestinal mucosa becomes strongly supplied with blood, which results in a healthy stimulation of the entire area.

Katherine P., 72, came into my office after a colonoscopy. "My doctor told me that diverticuli had formed on my intestinal walls. He said not to worry because he could always operate if I were to develop any symptoms. Do you know how to prevent more of them from forming?" I suggested the kind of urine therapy described above and the development was stopped.

Dysbacteria

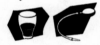

The first signs of a disrupted intestinal flora are belching, gas, intermittent constipation, and diarrhea. The so-called shigella can be contracted by anyone during vacation (from water or food), through flies, or from contact with excrement. The drinking of urine in the morning and small enemas (about 10 cc) at night, which are retained inside the intestine, help against the infection.

> **Tom H., 6, primary school student,** was
> brought to me by his mother because he had
> diarrhea. A stool test showed dysbacteria,
> which I treated as outlined above. After a
> week Tom was healthy and full of energy.

Hemorrhoids

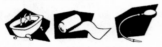

To eat meat while having itchy and bleeding hemorrhoids is a deadly sin. When the bleeding of the hemorrhoids has stopped, a sitz bath in moderately warm
tub water, with a collection of daily urine added, can
help. Afterward, rinse with lukewarm water. During
the night the bothersome hemorrhoids can be treated
with a gauze pad or tampon that has been soaked in
urine and placed in the crease between the buttocks.
Enemas (5 cc of fluid that stays within the rectum)
can be used also until the irritation has diminished.

Hypoactive pancreas

This problem cannot be treated with urine alone.
This condition frequently puts pressure on the heart
and lungs (interfering with breathing) and can cause

constipation and a bloated abdomen. Helpful in these cases are enemas with a small amount of urine (from 5 cc to 20 cc). They can be done several times daily (later in the treatment decrease to one every other evening and after six weeks only once a week). In addition, you can massage the abdomen clockwise with fresh urine for ten minutes in the morning. There is no need for rinsing, since it does not cause an odor when the liquid is completely rubbed in.

Intestinal disorders (ulcerative colitis/ Crohn's disease)

Urine therapists use small enemas, with the contents remaining within the intestine, to treat inflammatory intestinal disorders (either acute or chronic, such as Crohn's disease). Since the intestine is already irritated prior to the start of the treatment, therapists usually start with small units of 10 cc and often add a few drops of sunflower oil. With very weak or pain-sensitive patients the treatment should be performed every two days. For all other patients it should be done each day. The volume of the enemas should be increased every day until it finally reaches 40 cc. Other remedies may be added to the enemas as well, such as forta flower, multiplasan oil, or colibiogen, to help build up the intestinal mucosa. However, the decision to make additions must be made by the therapist.

Kidney infection

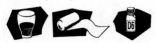

This extremely painful illness has two different forms. In acute cases back pain, swollen eyes, pressure and pain around the heart, and rising blood pressure point to a kidney infection. Prior to recommending oral urine therapy (in this case by the spoonful), it needs to be determined whether pus can be detected in the urine. If pus is present urine cannot be used in its pure form, only in the homeopathic form. Warm urine wraps (on the back at the level of the kidneys) can ease the pain and the infection at night. In case of a chronic infection (in most cases associated with edema in the feet and legs) the fresh urine can be used for drinking (but prior testing should be done). For the chronic ailment the following therapy is called for: One week of urine fasting (see the section entitled "A Quick Course in Treating Yourself") is a good introduction to the urine treatment. Ingest one sip of urine with each urination. After two weeks the treatment should be halted for one week. During this phase apply urine wraps every other day.

David N., 19, locksmith, complained of excruciating pain when he entered my office. He had an acute kidney infection, but with the aforementioned therapy the pain was gone after three days.

Kidney stones

The reason for this extremely painful illness is an abnormal elevation of uric acid levels in the blood serum. Gout is a good example of this process. If a kidney stone moves into the ureter it will cause severe pain. The pain can be eased through acupuncture in the ear. And then there is the horse cure in which a bottle of champagne, a bottle of beer, and half a liter of urine are mixed together and drunk in a shotgunlike fashion (or at least as fast as possible). The effect: The alcohol will ease the pain and the fluid impetus can flush the stone out.

If one does not like this brutal approach, one should use urine in a homeopathic way (every hour). One should drink an extremely large amount of fluid as well (it does not matter what kind). Everyone who has had a stone should expect another one. Recommended diet: a little fish; no innards; no cauliflower, spinach, or tomatoes; no alcohol or coffee, but lots of salads and juices instead.

Liver function disorders

Warning sign no. 1: If your stool shows a distinct yellow color, rather than a brown one, it indicates that your liver can no longer adequately break down fat. Your physician or naturopath will find elevated liver values in your blood. Therapy: Every night for four weeks a urine-soaked towel should be placed over the liver (in the right upper quadrant of the abdomen) and fixed with a second towel. This should remain in place overnight. The treatment may be discontinued after one week if the liver values have improved. In addition, the fat in the diet should be reduced and alcohol consumption should be terminated.

Sciatica/Lower back pain

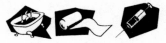

The best treatment is a bath with urine (about one liter of urine—collected over a week—in a bathtub full of water), rinsed off thoroughly afterward (no soap). Since this treatment also has a rather intense odor, hardly anyone will follow this advice. A very effective alternative is offered by the following method: The area of pain is injected with procaine and at night a cloth soaked in urine is wrapped around the hip and covered by a towel. It is left in place during sleep (in the morning there will be an odor). A shower without soap (preferably very warm) will eliminate the odor completely.

Paul A., 56, deliveryman, suffered from sciatica each fall, as soon as the weather turned colder. His physician's injection treatments did not agree with him anymore, and they had become less effective as well. Therefore he turned to me as a naturopath. I applied the therapy that I just mentioned and within three days Paul was symptom-free.

Umbilical colic

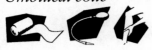

Sudden localized attacks around the umbilicus could point to an umbilical hernia. In this case most doctors would recommend surgery. Diffuse coliclike pain, though, can be eased with urine therapy. In these cases you should do the following: Twice a week insert a small urine enema (20 to 30 cc) into the rectum and leave it in place until it has been absorbed. In acute cases a urine compress can be placed over the umbilical area, and with each urination fresh urine can be rubbed in.

Vomiting

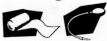

Urine therapy can only help against nausea if it is caused by nerves (meaning excitement, psychological stress, or overwork). Place warm rags soaked in urine on the upper belly (cover with a towel and place a hot water bottle on top of it). Keep the compress in place for about one hour and try to relax. Alternatively, every other day instill small enemas (20 to 30 cc) that remain in the colon. The drinking of urine in conjunction with a nervous stomach cannot be recommended.

Genital Area

Bladder infection

In the acute stage of a bladder infection drinking fluids is extremely important. The body needs lots of fluids, even if this seems absurd to the affected person who has to sit on the toilet for hours. In any event, you should contact your doctor or naturopath. The latter might treat the infection with an injection of your own urine, which has first been disinfected.

> **Lena F., 38, dental assistant,** had suffered frequently from bladder infections before she finally found her way to my office. "I always receive antibiotics and a few months later it happens again." For her acute complaints I used the injection therapy. After her urine had cleared, I recommended that she drink her own urine in the morning to boost her immune system and to protect her from recurrent complaints. Indeed, Lena has now been without an infection for two years.

Enlarged prostate gland

Many men have this problem and remain silent about it: Suddenly they have to get up every night and use the bathroom. The urine stream is not consistently strong anymore, but rather works like a plugged-up hose. Most often an enlarged prostate is the culprit.

> **Knut E., 54, plumber,** came to my office very worried: "I have problems when I pee. First of all it does not flow as well as it used
>
> *(cont.)*

to, and I also have to get up at two in the morning to use the bathroom. This is a big nuisance for me, since I have to get up at five in the morning anyway." In his examination the urologist detected an enlarged prostate. I recommended massaging the perineum with urine several times a day. In addition I also treated Knut twice a day with a small enema (the contents of which is retained within the intestine). I also recommended that he snack on pumpkin seeds and drink malva tea. In fact, he improved within a few weeks. The enlargement had regressed considerably.

Impotence

Massages with urine can work miracles for impotence if the problem is transient and not based on a medical dysfunction or a psychological blockage. Fresh urine should be rubbed around the pubic bone and on the back at the level of the pelvic bone. The drinking of morning urine on a regular basis can help also.

Menstrual problems

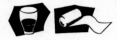

> **Melanie G., 17, high school student,** suffered from bad cramps on the first day of her menses: "My gynecologist could not find a plausible reason for it, but one year away from graduation I cannot afford to miss school so often for such a banality." I advised her to use warm urine compresses (dip a hand towel in urine and cover it with another towel; place a hot water bottle on top of it). I further recommended that she drink her urine on a regular basis or give herself a small enema (retained inside the intestine) every other day. First Melanie agreed to use the compresses and thanked me for the fast disappearance of her symptoms. Later she also started with oral urine therapy and has not had any problems for several months now.

Vagina

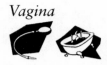

If the cause for vaginal complaints is not clear, a physician or naturopath should be consulted. In any case, it is beneficial to catch fresh urine and to irrigate the vagina with it (a kind of enema). Infections, itching, and small injuries or yeast infestations can be treated this way. In addition, sitz baths should be taken (one part chamomile tea to one part urine).

Vaginal discharge

To treat this complaint—which by the way is common for many women—an enema irrigation syringe from the drugstore is needed. At each urination fill the syringe with midstream urine and inject the liquid into the vagina. Alternatively, the urine can also be collected in a jar and used for the irrigation. The drinking of urine in the morning is a beneficial supportive measure.

Legs/Feet

Athlete's foot (Candida albicans)

Whether in a swimming pool or in a dressing room, anybody can easily contract the fungal infection athlete's foot. The treatment can be long and difficult. Nystatin (available as a powder or as an ointment) is one treatment. Urine therapy can also offer fantastic support. The affected foot should be soaked for ten minutes in the morning and at night in urine that has been collected over several days. Afterward the remaining fluid should be massaged into the skin. (If you can bear the odor, please don't rinse.) During the night, gauze pads soaked in urine can be placed inside socks. The socks should be made from cotton, be changed daily, and be washed in a washing machine with hot water (at least 60°C, 140°F). Within three days the foot should have recovered significantly.

Circulation problems

Sensations of coldness, numbness, or pallor in arms or legs can be helped with a massage of the corresponding extremities with older urine (although this will smell, its penetrating effect is very beneficial). Even more effective is a urine massage, if prior to it the extremities have been rubbed with sisal gloves in a circular motion moving toward the heart. In this way urine will be absorbed even better and the odor will be kept to a minimum.

These steps should not be applied to venous circulatory problems like varicose veins or stasis.

Philip K., 61, bank clerk, came to my office: "I have varicose veins. I heard that massages with a brush can help against them." I told him how dangerous this can be (it can trigger bleeding) and recommended a cold water-jet treatment starting from his toes and moving upward toward the hips, as well as cold urine compresses. His varicose veins did not disappear, of course, but the circulation was stimulated through the urine and Philip had no more pain in his legs during the night.

Frostbite

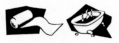

War veterans might remember the healing effect of a urine rub on frostbitten hands and feet. Compresses, which are used through the night, heal these painful wounds extremely quickly.

Ingrid W., 40, registered nurse, came to my office after her ski vacation. She had frost-bitten fingertips, which made her suffer with pain. I advised a urine bath. This is done by collecting fresh urine, preferably the morning one, in a small bowl. Carefully move the fingertips around in it. After one week Ingrid came back to me: "You won't believe it, the pain and the white spots, everything has disappeared. Once again I can move my fingers well and I have gone back to work."

Legs (open sores)

Through urine the healing does not start superficially with the formation of new skin, but the wound slowly closes up from the base. This takes longer but is far more effective, because new infections could possibly form underneath the skin otherwise.

Henry D., 83, lives with his daughter, who has cared for her father for many years. He had open leg sores and traditional medicine had long given up on him ("You just have to live with it"). When his daughter Betty read the first urine therapy book she gained hope again. She writes: "For years I had seen my father suffering. Then I persuaded him to try the urine therapy. Each morning he collected his urine and I soaked gauze pads in it." This, by the way, is very important: Always use gauze from the drugstore, never use cotton balls. Cotton can get caught in open wounds and can cause infection. "Then I placed the pads over his wounds and bandaged his legs. Four weeks later I could already see a clear improvement. After three months the legs were completely healed; a true miracle."

Phlebitis

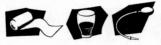

Before this illness can be treated it is absolutely important to exclude the danger of a thrombus or embolus. Talk to your physician about it. Cold urine compresses should then be used and exchanged frequently after they have warmed up. This should be done daily for about two hours. The oral intake of urine in the morning and urine-retention enemas at night support the healing process. The therapy ends when the phlebitis is completely healed.

Marie J., 67, came into my practice with phlebitis. Her doctor had prescribed medications for previous infections, but the package information of these drugs alarmed the patient. I suggested urine therapy to her and was surprised by her reaction: "You know, I've already thought about it myself. My mother used urine a lot for us six children. No matter if we had a sore throat, burned fingers, or wounds after small fights. I just didn't know for sure whether urine would help in my case." The infection indeed healed up within ten days. The patient now drinks her morning urine on a regular basis, so that the inflammation attacks won't repeat themselves.

Sprains

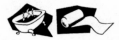

During the olden times of our grandmothers the village kids who had sprained their ankles would be told, "Stick your foot in the cow bucket." In it the urine of the livestock had been collected. Within a short time the pain would subside, and in most cases the swelling could be prevented also. A sprained wrist or foot still may be treated very well with urine. For this treatment you can collect your urine for the whole day. Let the fluid soak into the affected area for at least half an hour. If possible, do not shower afterward, but rather massage the rest of the urine into the skin. Cold wraps, which always should be exchanged after they have warmed up, are also very helpful.

Varicose veins

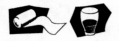

When varicose veins begin to show clearly underneath the skin or to protrude, it is time to do something about them. Varicose veins are not only a nuisance and sometimes painful (cramps in the calf), they can be also dangerous since they raise the possibility of a thrombosis. Of great importance: Under no circumstance treat varicose veins with massages or heat. On the contrary cold showers can be helpful.

Marion M., 43, waitress, writes: "In your book about urine therapy you also gave recommendations about varicose veins. I alternate cold showers with cold urine compresses, drink my morning urine daily, and during my last fall vacation I did a week of urine fasting. The result: The swelling stopped, the big blue clots have regressed. I don't have any more cramping in my lower legs (but I have also started to take magnesium), and I have regained the same strength I had fifteen years ago."

Skin

Acne

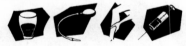

The ground rule for each treatment of acute or chronic acne is: The treatment will take as long as the skin symptoms have existed. This treatment normally consists of three steps. First a six-day urine fast, then an oral therapy with morning midstream urine taken daily over six weeks (if you cannot make the decision to drink your urine you can use retention enemas or urine injections performed by a therapist). During the entire treatment time (four to eight weeks may go by before you see successful results) each fresh urine should be massaged into the face.

Bedsores

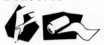

Cupping with alcohol and frequent repositioning are the only possibilities for preventing a decubitus (bedsore). If one occurs anyway the old adage applies: Miracles don't happen overnight. This is also true for bedsores and their healing process. The regeneration of the skin is only possible from the bottom of the wound upward and takes time and patience. However, if it regenerates from the base up it is more durable and will not get infected easily. Urine wraps and the cleaning of the wounds have proven beneficial in these cases. Both should be done with fresh urine only. The wraps should be applied cool and should always be changed as soon they have warmed up.

Burns

Have you ever burned yourself on a hot iron or a hot lid? This would be a good opportunity to try out the effects of your urine. Wet the area with some of your fresh urine, which you carefully rub in. This will keep you from getting burn blisters, which not even ice-cold water can achieve (though otherwise it is a very good remedy for burns).

Diaper rash

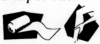

Diaper rash does not have anything to do with wet diapers, as the advertisements want you to believe. This would mean that generations of babies before the development of moisture barriers had to suffer from tormenting pains. Babies develop diaper rashes either because their mothers have eaten an irritating food and have passed it on through the breast milk or because the baby itself has an intolerance to a particular food (a common example: oranges).

As long as the rash consists only of inflamed skin the application of urine to the affected area can be very helpful. Try out cotton diapers for a change and you will see how quickly the redness will disappear. When there are open areas on the baby's buttocks: Discontinue urine treatments.

Eczema

Mary L. was only nine months old when her mother brought her to my office. The little one had eczema on her fingers, which looked similar to neurodermatitis. However, every allergy test indicated that neurodermatitis was not the cause. The mother did not want to treat the baby with cortisone cream any longer. Since such a small child cannot be convinced to drink urine (which would be recommended to balance the body), I advised the mother to give Mary small enemas (5 cc in a syringe without a needle) and to moisten the affected areas with urine (which could be achieved with a recently wetted diaper, as long as the baby wears a cotton diaper).

Mary's mother carried out my advice. After two days the child stopped scratching her itching eczema (since the itch had vanished) and the skin started to heal up. Mary is fifteen months old now and has had no further complaints in the last three months.

Fistula

These pimplelike infections underneath the skin with a large duct that drains the secretion to the outside are revolting but not serious. Fistulae generally appear in areas in which the skin is very thin and exposed to constant friction. If they are weeping wounds and the infection spreads to the surrounding area, they can become very unpleasant. A treatment that anybody can perform is the urine instillation. In a 10 cc syringe, mix 5 cc of fresh urine with 2 cc of arnica tincture. If the tip of the needle is too wide, a hypodermic needle could be used. The needle's tip should be broken off, so it will not puncture the inside wall of the duct. The urine-arnica solution should then be injected into the duct. Most of the solution will run out again immediately, the rest will be absorbed. It will suppress the infection and activate the immune system. The therapy should be repeated every day until the symptoms subside. If, in the future, even the smallest tension shows up underneath the skin, one or two treatments with the syringe should be enough to stop the fistula in its early stages.

Herpes

This is an infection that usually appears periodically on the lips, when the immune system has been weakened or when the psyche is under stress. Another area that can be affected is the genital area. The application of fresh urine helps in all cases (if possible with the appearance of the first signs). Afterward, wash your hands thoroughly, which is important not because of the urine, but due to the possibility of an autoinfection. This means you could spread the small blisters from the lips all the way to the chin. In the genital area a urine-soaked gauze pad can be used overnight. In addition to this treatment one should also follow through with a basic urine therapy (six weeks of morning urine orally). This could lead to an internal change of the body.

> **Mary Ann W., 31, actress,** was absolutely annoyed when she came to see me: "I break out with herpes on my lips over and over again. This is very troublesome since the makeup person cannot always mask over it. Every time we have a premiere coming up I can be certain that at least twenty-four

hours before the big day my lips will start to break out." I explained to her how the basic urine therapy works. I also told her that besides her psychological stress about debuts, her increased exhaustion would play a role in her recurrent infection as well, since the actors rehearse for many hours before the big event, which puts a lot of stress on the immune system. And indeed, Mary Ann got through the next premiere without a fat lip. The basic urine therapy was successful.

Infections

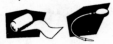

The different treatment methods for infections of the eye, inside the ears, and in the throat are listed under the corresponding phrases. External infections on different parts of the body can be well treated with cold compresses, which should be changed after they have warmed up. For open wounds only fresh urine is recommended. For swelling underneath the skin old urine shows a better result because it penetrates deeper into the skin. If the infections turn into chronic ones (that is, they return repeatedly), a small retention enema with about 10 cc of urine should be used.

Insect bites

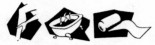

Scratching insect bites can cause infections. Not scratching, on the other hand, requires some will-power, which not everyone can come up with. The itch is too unpleasant, but it will disappear quickly after applying urine to the skin. The same is true for wasp stings. Should the area swell up anyway bathing the affected body part in a urine-water solution might help. (If the reaction is very extreme, you must consult your physician immediately, since you might be allergic to the wasp's poison.) Bee stings should be soaked in plain urine since it helps to draw out the stinger (keep it up for at least half an hour). This makes the removal of the stinger with tweezers easier. Finally, you should cover the sting with a urine compress to reduce the existing swelling.

Itching

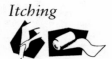

As mentioned earlier with insect bites, urine can help to reduce the itch. You can apply it directly or with a compress, which is applied overnight (or for several hours) and is fixed to the body. Within a few hours the symptoms should disappear.

> **Michelle L., 23, mother of two-year-old Lisa,** wrote to me: "We were close to Berlin at a lake and in the evening the mosquitoes were attacking us. When we got home Lisa was already dead tired, but could not go to sleep because the mosquito bites on her back were tormenting her. I remembered your recipe and asked her to pee in her potty, in which I had placed a cotton diaper. I wrung it out and placed it on her naked back (the room was warm anyway). After just half an hour Lisa was doing better and she finally fell asleep.

Jellyfish stings

When a jellyfish makes contact with the skin a burning rash appears. Quick relief can be obtained with your own urine. Simply collect the urine on a tissue and place it immediately on the burning areas. The burning will subside within half an hour.

Ellen M., 31, wrote about her experience at the beach during her vacation with her three children. Timmy was playing by himself in the shallow water when suddenly he started to cry. Ellen wrote, "I ran to him and saw that a jellyfish was hanging onto his lower leg. I took it off and brought him back to the beach. Timmy cried with pain. I ran back to our blanket, grabbed some tissues, and carried the child into the dunes. There I told him to pee, but he was too agitated. So I asked his brother, who is two years older, to pee. I had learned from your first book on urine therapy that for external injuries without bleeding another person's urine is as effective for healing as the injured person's own. Half an hour later all signs of the jellyfish burn had disappeared.

Urine can be helpful also if you step on a sea urchin. You need to bathe your foot in pure urine until the quills can be pushed out of the skin. Then you can pull them out completely with tweezers.

Kaposi's sarcoma

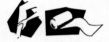

It is said that the appearance of Kaposi's sarcoma (sicklelike tissue tumors under the skin) can be slowed with the help of urine therapy (every day fresh urine should be rubbed on the affected area). Compresses applied overnight also help. These skin lesions often can be found in connection with AIDS.

Psoriasis

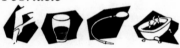

Fresh urine should be rubbed on the affected areas or (if they are too sensitive) should be swabbed on. In addition, a basic urine therapy is recommended. If you cannot drink the urine, insert 20 to 30 cc of urine rectally at night, which must be completely absorbed by the intestine. Urine baths, with a few handfuls of sea salt added if possible and hot enough for one to stay in for fifteen minutes, should also heal the skin and reduce the itching immediately.

Scars

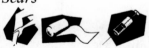

Scars—especially in the facial area—can be rather disturbing. To make the skin more pliable and to help it blend into the surrounding normal skin, the scars should be massaged with morning urine. Practitioners can also try injections directly underneath the skin to stimulate the healing process. Compresses fixed onto the scar at night can also speed up healing (this treatment takes about 4 weeks).

Shingles

> **Albert H., 46, technical graphic designer,** had been under stress for months. He constantly had to work overtime at the office and, moreover, he was building his own house. Free time had become a foreign word to him. When he came to my office this big, strong man was suddenly very quiet: "I can't see it but my wife tells me that I have an open wound under my shoulder blade, which drains fluid. Sometimes it hurts, too." I examined him and found the beginning of shingles the size of a silver dollar.
>
> In this early stage shingles can still be treated well with urine therapy. I recommended fresh urine compresses, which should be held in place at night with a

bandage. I also urgently advised the patient to start with a relaxation therapy like yoga or autogenous training.

I had to tell Albert: "If you don't learn right away how to relax completely for short periods of time, your body will start to go on strike." Since Albert's first visit his family has moved into the new house and the patient has started a relaxation program to regain his fitness. Luckily we stopped the shingles in its early stages.

Stinging nettle burns

The stung area should be swabbed with fresh urine immediately. The more quickly the procedure is done the more successful it will be.

John T., 24, student, amateur ornithologist, walks through the forests and fields on the weekends to watch birds. When the goal is to keep his feathered friends within his view, he does not show much consideration for himself. He wrote to me: "In your
(cont.)

book I read the tip about fresh urine for nettle stings. After I ran into a field of stinging nettles (one should not look only through the binoculars), I tried rubbing urine onto both of my legs. After minutes the burning had vanished. When it reappeared in the evening I repeated the therapy again. I have never gotten better so fast after burning myself on stinging nettle."

Sunburn

Drive through the night and the next morning you are on the beach in the sun. This is a dangerous way to start a vacation. If you fall asleep on the beach, you can get a very bad sunburn since the water reflects the sun especially intensely. There are many sunburn lotions on the market, but not all are tolerated by sensitive skin. A simple household remedy: Urine mixed with olive oil placed on the affected areas and left overnight. In bad cases of sunburn repeat several times.

Harold M., 34, taxi driver, drove six hours in his own car from Munich to Livorno in Italy. He writes: "Because of the children I drove all night. They slept in the car, and the next day I continued on without a break. We went to the beach. While the kids went swimming I fell asleep. Four hours later I woke up like a red tomato. My whole back was burned including the backs of my legs. That evening in our room I remembered a remedy from your first urine therapy book. I mixed olive oil, which I got from our landlady, with fresh urine and rubbed it several times on my skin. Next morning, the burning sensation was already gone and my daughter told me that I was not as red anymore. I could even go swimming that day despite the salt water, though I spent the next few days in the shade. My skin did not peel. I now gladly pass on this advice, which I owe to your book.

Superficial wounds

> **Sylvia D., salesclerk,** had a lot of fun with her new kittens, but also received many scratches during their play. She wrote, "This was a good opportunity to test your claims about the fast healing of such wounds. And sure enough, when I rubbed my hands with urine, they looked better after only one night. Within three days all the scratches had disappeared, except for the new ones my kittens had given me, of course."

Body

Anemia

Pallor, weakness, and fatigue can point to a possible anemia (not enough red blood cells).This should definitely be diagnosed by a physician or naturopath, since the reason for this disorder could also be more severe.

Nina H., 17, gymnast, came to me after her doctor had diagnosed her with anemia. "He prescribed iron pills, which my stomach can't tolerate. On the other hand, I do want to do something about my weakness, since I want to graduate this year and I don't feel strong enough for the tests." First, I explained to her that she could substitute for iron tablets with beet juice, fish, and once a week, liver. I also told her about the possibility of treating her with urine therapy and recommended a basic urine therapy. Since she absolutely ruled out the option of drinking urine, I prescribed a retention enema with around 20 cc of urine, which remains in the colon. After six weeks she had improved markedly.

Arteriosclerosis

Calcium deposits in the arteries can make the circulation very difficult and can also harm the body's oxygen supply, which in the end will ruin the metabolism of the cells. The first noticeable signs are circulation disturbances in arms and legs. Here one should begin with urine massages. Urine penetrates deeply under the skin and promotes better circulation. At the same time the drinking of urine in the morning should become a habit. In this way a turnaround of the body can be achieved.

Andre K., 67, retired, suffered for years with arteriosclerosis. The circulation problems in his arms caused him both numbness and pain. A few weeks after he started the recommended oral urine therapy in conjunction with massages, the pain ceased. Later, his numbness subsided also.

Blood pressure (high)

See *Hypertension.*

Bruises

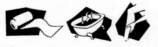

If somebody has had a bad accident and suffers from bruises, friends like to offer comfort: "You were lucky that nothing worse happened." But anybody who has had bruises in the past would disagree strongly because the pain is quite severe. Start the treatment for the hematoma early by rubbing it down with urine, which can prevent swelling of the bruise.

> **Steven C., 29, bicycle courier,** had been hit by a car in a driveway and had bruised his hip. "This really hurt badly. At night I could hardly sleep because of the pain (How can one lie down comfortably with such an injury?). Then I started flipping through the pages in your book and I tried the urine wraps. I soaked a towel in urine, let it cool down, and fixed it with a scarf to my hip. The next morning the swelling had already gone down and with urine massages the worst was over within three days."

Candidiasis (yeast infection)

Yeast infections on the feet, in the mouth, and on the scalp are easy to detect. Much more difficult is the question of whether yeast is growing in the intestine. Only a stool sample that has been sent off to a reference lab can give a definite answer. A simple test for yeast can be done by anybody: Let your urine sit for twenty-four hours (a jar with a lid is the best, since an odor will develop otherwise). If you detect yellow flakes you should consult a physician or a naturopath to further investigate the matter.

See *Athlete's Foot, Bloating/Flatulence, Scalp, Thrush,* and *Vagina* for specific treatment methods in detail.

Chicken pox

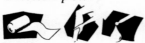

Chicken pox is the most common childhood disease. It usually starts with blisterlike spots on the chest and then spreads to the face, the arms, and the genital area. They appear in phases every three to four days. They quickly crust over and itch severely. Sometimes the illness goes along with a fever (treat with urine wraps on the lower legs) or with headaches (apply fresh urine to the temples, neck, or behind the ears). If the rash has shown up inside the ears urine eardrops can be helpful (the ear should be plugged in this case with a cotton ball soaked in oil). In addition, fresh urine can be applied directly to the pustules and should ease the itching within three days. This is important since scratching of the sores can lead to scars. The child is no longer contagious after the last spots have crusted over.

Cramps

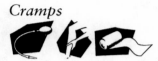

The reason for these abdominal pains could be indigestion, gas, or menstrual problems. Most often an enema (1 to 2 liters urine) will help immediately. If the pain is caused by the kidney or gallbladder a warm, circular massage with urine can be a good complementary therapy. This coliclike pain, however, needs to be explored further by a physician or naturopath, since the causes could be rather dangerous. If the patient is sensitive to touch, towels soaked in urine and kept warm by a hot water bottle placed on the stomach can help.

Diabetes

This disease, which is commonly called "sugar," can indeed be detected through the urine: It is sweeter than the urine of a person with normal blood sugar values. In Japan, even nowadays, it is common practice to prescribe the basic urine therapy against diabetes. The Japanese are convinced that the sugar in the urine will remind the body to release more insulin from the pancreas.

Carla F., 42, educator, was shocked when her doctor informed her that her blood sugar values were elevated. She told me in my office: "On the positive side, he tried to comfort me because the values were only slightly elevated. The reason his news frightened me so much was that my father died from complications of diabetes. Of course I am willing to change my diet. But is there anything else I can do?" I talked with Carla about urine therapy and also recommended to her that in the future she needs to listen to her body carefully, watching weight and exercise, but also getting enough rest. After being in my treatment for over a year, drinking her urine every day, and doing exercises, she has maintained her normal weight and her blood sugar levels have remained within the normal values.

Dog bite

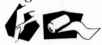

Do not hesitate for long: Place the wound immediately under the urine stream, massage the fluid in, and rinse it. In this way the urine will penetrate deeply into the injured skin. A loose urine-soaked bandage during the night should improve the wound significantly within twenty-four hours. If puncture wound is present: Check whether your tetanus immunization is up to date, or whether you need a booster shot. And with a dog bite, of course, there is always the possibility of rabies. Do not take these injuries lightly but consult a doctor immediately.

Edema

Water accumulation in the tissue of the feet and lower legs is very common in the summertime. Urine massages (you may use old urine) can be a beneficial remedy. Everybody who has a tendency toward edema should also do something in general to correct this disposition. My suggestion: fasting with urine for one week to ten days and afterward, the regular drinking of urine in the morning.

Extremity pain

If someone feels like "every bone in the body" is hurting, the pain can be due to different causes. The problem could be overexertion (too much exercise after a rest period), tension, or an infection associated with a fever. Collect the urine from an entire day. Rub it on the painful points at night and afterward take a warm bath to which the remaining urine is added.

> **Martin B., 28, retailer,** writes: "During the winter months I always become a little lazy, watch a lot of TV, and don't move around much. When the weather improves in the spring we start to get out in our rowboats and in the evening I often have pain in my arms. In your urine therapy book I read the recipe for aches and pains. I tried it out and I am absolutely fervent about it. Afterward I soak in warm water and go to bed immediately. This is also a great remedy for the first signs of a flu. The next morning everything feels much better."

Fever

There is no reason to fight fever in a radical way, since it is a rather beneficial reaction of the immune system designed to fight off an infection. A higher risk exists in babies and toddlers, who can develop a fever more rapidly. Also, when the fever rises very high and lasts for a long time, it could weaken the patient. In these cases—our grandmothers already knew this—cold wraps around the calf muscle will help. If these wraps are not only soaked in lukewarm water but also in cooled urine, the body temperature will not only come down but a stimulus will be given to the immune system as well.

Betty K., 29, mother of three-year-old Katherine, confirmed my experience in a letter: "Our Katherine catches a cold very easily and develops a high fever. I got the tip about the cold wraps from your earlier book on urine therapy and half a year ago I tried it for the first time. The effect was amazing: After just three hours (I had changed the wraps continuously) her temperature had dropped from 40°C (104.9°F) to 38.5°C (101.3°F). The next cold epidemic in her daycare left Katherine untouched for the first time."

Furunculosis (boils)

Fresh urine should be applied with cotton Q-tips or directly onto developing acute furuncles (at any time during the day). Anybody suffering from a chronic case of furuncles can try to attune the body with the help of basic urine therapy.

Gout

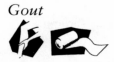

More men suffer from gout than women, since this illness is caused by an increased urine acid level, which happens in men more often. The reason for the elevation lies within the diet (too much protein). A crystalline sediment of salts causes swelling and pain in the joints. The metabolism is hyperacidic. A diet change (among other things avoid alcohol, coffee, and meat) in this case is unavoidable. Acute painful areas can be treated directly with fresh urine (also with older urine) or can be treated with a urine wrap overnight.

Hormone imbalances

Young women especially, who might have taken birth control pills for many years, suffer from hormone imbalances (such as disturbances in the menstrual cycle, hair loss, weight gain, etc.). But a bad illness or psychosomatic disorder can wreak havoc with the hormone balance as well. Here, urine therapy serves well. It sends an impulse to the body to balance itself. And it has one big advantage: It is without any side effects. In severe cases a combination therapy of five days of urine fasting followed by a course of basic urine therapy is recommended.

Miriam G., 30, translator, arrived in my office with these complaints: "Six months after my wedding I stopped taking the pill because we wished for a child. Instead of getting pregnant, I've gained weight, have developed oily hair and pimples, and my period is no longer regular." For thirteen years this young woman had taken the pill and incapacitated her natural hormone functioning. I explained to her that we had to rebuild it slowly and recommended the combination therapy. She followed the treatment in an exemplary manner and week after week her symptoms decreased. Six months later, Miriam was pregnant.

Hot flashes

See *Menopause*.

Hypertension

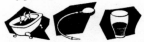

Urine is effective against hypertension (levels that are continually above 160/100 mm Hg) only when used as an ongoing therapy. This means urine fasting (10 days) once a year followed by drinking the midstream urine every morning (or, alternatively, taking an indwelling urine enema of about 40 cc every other day). After a month one pauses for a consecutive month until the levels have stabilized. The symptoms (lack of interest, dizziness, nausea) are almost the same as for a blood pressure that is too low. Recommended for hypertension are moderately warm baths with urine added, which will influence the microcirculation and should be taken at night before going to bed. For a low blood pressure the baths can be nicely warm. Afterward, take a cold shower to stimulate your circulation.

Gretchen T., 67, tried this remedy for hypertension after she came to my practice with relatively high readings. "Is there still a treatment for me? Or do I have to live with the beta blockers now?" she asked me. I told her about the aforementioned treatment and persuaded her furthermore to go on a moderate diet, which would make her lose one pound a week (the slower the weight reduction, the longer it will last). Gretchen has lost thirteen pounds and her blood pressure is back to normal levels.

Immune deficiency

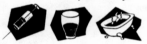

If you are constantly battling lingering infections it is time to do something about the weakness of your immune system. It is best to fight it in multiple ways: A naturopath can achieve a lot with self-transfusion and urine injections. In addition, one week of urine fasting should follow a basic urine therapy. Every week a bath with urine added to the water stimulates the body externally.

Infection (flulike)

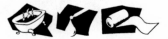

In the evening take a bath with very warm water and add a liter of collected urine. Go to bed immediately afterward (cover yourself well). This is a very old household remedy. To sweat out an infection is possible. Nose (drops), ears (drops), and chest (chest wraps against cough) could be treated as well. And another tip: While lying down, let 5 cc of urine run into your nose. If it burns too much, make a 1:1 mixture with chamomile tea. The fluid will spread over the entire pharyngeal and sinus cavity and has an infection-fighting effect.

Joint pain

See *Arthritis* or *Arthrosis*.

Lack of energy

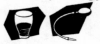

Do you feel exhausted, are you always tired, and do you have a hard time concentrating? If so you'd better get used to the basic urine therapy, the drinking of morning midstream urine in a six-week rhythm. If you really cannot bring yourself to do it try starting with just one sip with each urination. Or, alternatively, you can try indwelling enemas (about 20 to 30 cc in the colon). These need to be taken every other day. If your condition gets really bad a week of urine fasting is a good remedy for getting your body and immune system back in shape.

Leukopenia

If you have swollen lymph nodes and you experience a recurring fever, you should consult a physician or naturopath immediately. You might have leukopenia, an immune system deficiency characterized by a low white blood cell count. Oral urine therapy can be a supportive treatment. You can drink your morning midstream urine regularly or can use a indwelling enema every two days.

Sophie B., 17, student, had suffered from a severe, infectious pneumonia when her doctor diagnosed her with leukopenia. I recommended the basic urine therapy since, besides raising her white blood cell count, I expected it to enhance her immune system. And indeed, after only three weeks her levels were significantly above the minimum count of 5,000/mm^3. Sophie felt better overall, and she had gotten used to the morning drink. She decided to continue it: "I never want to get as sick again as I did after the pneumonia. Therefore I will do everything I can do for my immune system."

Menopause

Between the ages of forty-five and fifty every woman will eventually experience menopause, the so-called change of life. The end of menstruation, that is, of fertility, is connected with many hormonal changes within the body. Conventional medicine tries to take the easy way out: It substitutes for natural hormones with hormone replacement tablets. This of course means that the body will terminate its own hormone production even faster than normal. Depression, mood swings, sleep disorders, hot flashes—all of these belong to the farewell to womanhood, just as acne, weight disturbances, and changeable moods during puberty marked the beginning of womanhood.

Anita L., 49, housewife, came to my office one day: "I've already seen a gynecologist about my complaints and he wanted to prescribe hormones. I thought that I'd rather look for an alternative treatment." In fact, some of the homeopathic remedies and urine therapy can help in this case. For the menopausal years a modified drink therapy is recommended. The morning midstream urine should be drunk until the

> symptoms subside. Afterward one may
> pause for six weeks. If the symptoms reap-
> pear one should drink urine only on the
> acute days. Anita followed my advice and
> today she says: "Since I began drinking
> urine I seldom have mood changes or hot
> flashes anymore.

Actually, the information that the urine gives to the
body is not only of a physical nature. Emotional conditions can also be changed with its help.

Morning sickness

Urine therapy against morning sickness? Sounds like
a paradox but it really works for women who are
already used to drinking urine. If someone feels nau-
seated already it is hard to get accustomed to a difficult new practice. But the inexperienced can still reap
some of urine's benefits by using a homeopathic form
(four times daily).

Mumps

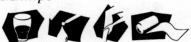

Except for warm compresses, folk medicine had no
real treatment against this childhood illness that can

affect adults as well. The disease is an infection of the parotid gland and oral cavity, which often coincides with a fever and can affect either one or both sides. The "fat cheeks" are the most obvious sign. This is always accompanied by fever, which can be relieved by cool urine wraps on the lower legs. The illness itself can be soothed through urine gargling, urine eardrops, and urine massages and compresses on the affected side.

Obesity

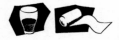

After many different diets even hard-core hunger diets don't work anymore. Urine therapy could enhance weight loss. Start with drinking your urine (daily if possible) and once a week do a whole-body urine pack. This is done the following way: Spread a cotton blanket on your bed, cover it with a plastic sheet, and place a sheet on top of it that has been soaked in urine. Lie on it and wrap each layer around you (it is good to have help). At the end cover yourself with another blanket and stay under it for two hours (you might even fall asleep). Afterward you can rinse your body off with a warm shower (since an unpleasant odor will have appeared). Using soap is not necessary.

Andrea P., 34, salesclerk in a bakery, was about 30 kg (66 pounds) overweight when she came to me: "Name any kind of diet, I have tried them all and even lost some weight. But I've always gained more weight back afterward. And now no diet has an effect anymore. My husband says that based on what I eat and drink he doesn't see how I can be so obese." I recommended urine therapy for her and a division diet. Andrea kept up with it and has lost 23 kg so far. She wants to continue.

Osteoporosis

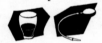

This illness can be a side effect of the hormone changes experienced during menopause or it can be hereditary. Osteoporosis means a slow decalcification of the bone, which leads to a predisposition for breaks with prolonged healing times. Practitioners can counter these results with a whole catalog of actions: gymnastics and swimming (active movement), which are just as important as a complete diet; a calcium supplement (preferably a homeopathic one, so that the body's natural calcium absorption gets activated again); and a continuous urine therapy (urine fasting, six weeks of drinking urine, six weeks of 30 cc enemas every other evening). These measures can bring this negative development to a halt and eventually may even lead to a reversal.

Barbara F., 48, optician, came to my office after an accident. She had broken her ankle during a ski vacation, which also led to a discovery by her doctors. "They told me that I have the beginning of osteoporosis and prescribed to me high dosages of calcium. Is this all I can do against it?" I recommended the combination therapy that I mentioned above. Indeed, Barbara's calcium levels have stabilized and she has been able to keep her illness in check.

Paralysis

Accidents, strokes, and different diseases can lead to paralysis. Urine massages can be an effective complementary treatment. First the affected area should be dry brushed (be careful, the skin can be very sensitive) and afterward massaged with urine that has been collected in a capped bottle for several days.

Helen H., 73, describes her experience with urine therapy in a letter to me: "My husband, who is five years older than I am, had suffered from a stroke a year ago with a paralysis of the left arm. He could not lift the arm and he could only move his fingers a little. After the rehabilitation he had to go to the physiotherapist. In addition, I massaged his arm with urine twice a day. Within six months his symptoms subsided to a degree that his disability was hardly noticeable. His doctor was very much surprised by his fast recovery, which he had not expected in a seventy-eight-year-old man.

Phantom pain

It's worth a try, you have nothing to lose: The basic urine therapy (six weeks of drinking the urine in the morning) can attune the body by sending out small nerve impulses to the amputated body parts that send and receive signals.

Rheumatism

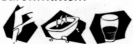

Hereditary predisposition is not the only reason for this illness. Further contributing factors are a hyper-acidic diet, lack of exercise, and cold weather. A change in diet is necessary: almost no fat, little or no meat, alcohol, white flour, or white sugar. Instead, eat lots of fruits and vegetables and use brown sugar or, even better, honey. Urine therapy can be used for rheumatism in multiple ways: Acute painful areas can be rubbed down with urine, a weekly urine bath (very hot for fifteen minutes) is beneficial, and urine fasting once a year can be helpful. The fundamental change of the body can be supported by the basic urine therapy. After three months of basic urine therapy a week-long break should follow.

Scarlet fever

The symptoms are a sore throat accompanied by tonsillitis (the throat looks burning red), fever, vomiting, abdominal pain due to swollen lymph glands, strawberry-like spots on a coated tongue, and finally a rash, which begins at the neck and moves down slowly over the entire body. In the old times the bed linen of a patient was burned and the children were often placed on the isolation floor of a hospital.

Today, thirty years later, scarlet fever presents itself in a comparatively harmless form. After the initial incidence there is usually a recovering interval followed soon after by a second illness.

> **Florian, 8,** was lucky since his mother, Irene D., 42, knew about urine therapy. She wrote to me: "My mother treated us with urine and helped us in this way with our childhood diseases. Your book brought back a lot of my mother's knowledge. I first let Florian gargle with a urine-chamomile mixture, gradually changing to pure urine. I also applied urine to his rash because he was complaining about the itching. Amazingly, after two days my boy felt so much better."

Sore muscles

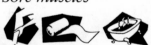

Have you ever played a team sport with friends after not having played for five years? Did you ever take a massive hike during vacation? The price for such actions is usually sore muscles and strains (working at a computer monitor can also cause soreness). Urine massages help wonderfully (the urine is collected over days in a capped bottle). Work the skin first with a dry brush then massage in the fluid. Urine wraps (overnight) can also break up tensions.

Thomas G., 28, clerk, writes to me in a letter: "In the last few years I have really gotten out of shape behind my desk. When a friend invited me to play soccer one Sunday morning, it seemed like a good idea to me. In the evening, however, I could hardly move and it did not seem like a good idea at all anymore. Remembering your book, I started to collect my urine and took a bath the next evening with one liter of urine in the bath water. Afterward, I rubbed my aching thighs with the urine. The next morning I felt so much better. To be safe, I massaged with urine again in the evening and was symptom-free on Wednesday."

Ulcerations

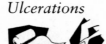

It is important to thoroughly clean the ulcers prior to the treatment. Next, place compresses that have been soaked in fresh warm urine on the ulcers and change them several times within the next two hours.

Especially in cases of open sores one should only use fresh and sterile urine. If the ulcer is located where it can be wetted directly by urine, that should be done. Within a week a clear, marked improvement should be noted.

> **Walter M., 32, goldsmith,** hurt himself with a tool. At the site of the wound an ulcer formed, which he showed to me: "My girlfriend thinks it should be lanced but I am afraid of having it done. That's the reason I came to you." Walter was not very enthusiastic about the possibility of using his own urine for the healing process, but finally agreed to it. After five days his ulcer had disappeared.

Whooping cough

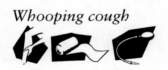

> **Stephanie, 5,** had whooping cough a year ago. Her mother Maria F., 32, wrote about it in a letter to me: "The nights were especially gruesome. Steffi coughed and coughed.
> *(cont.)*

One night I went to the bookshelf and looked for your book, since I remembered that there was something in it about whooping cough. I tried it out. The very next night my daughter could sleep for six hours again, for the first time in a week. I was so happy!"

The following treatment helped the child: Rub the chest with urine (you may add two drops of menthol oil), or apply chest wraps during the night with this mixture. In the morning and at night administer a small enema (5 cc), which will stay in the colon until it is absorbed. Instill nosedrops (1:1 urine/chamomile solution). In cases of high fever cold urine wraps on the lower leg muscles can be very helpful.

Yeast infections

See *Candidiasis*.

Emotional Disorders

Anxiety, panic/tranquilizer

Hormones are excreted from the body along with the urine, among them the calming melatonin. That is why a six-week-long basic urine therapy can effectively control anxiety. Also, in cases of anxiety the mild healing method should be favored over the psychopharmaceutical treatment.

Fear/Fear suppressor

Survivors of airplane crashes or shipwrecks who had to survive without water, and therefore started to drink their own urine, were the first who made an astounding discovery: Not only could they stop their tormenting thirst but they also found that their paniclike fear subsided. Experts agree that urine, with its melatonin content, has a calming effect.

Sleep disorder/Sleeping aid

Taking a bedtime enema (with 30 cc of urine that remains inside the body) every two days can relax the body. Taking a warm bedtime bath with one liter of urine added also has a calming effect. In addition to this: no food after seven P.M., a small walk, and possibly a glass of wine or a beer for relaxation. This is better than using sleeping pills, which can cause emotional dependency.

DIFFERENT COUNTRIES,
DIFFERENT CUSTOMS

The first written records of urine therapy are found in the ancient Egyptian *Ebers Papyrus* from about 1000 B.C. These deal mainly with the applications that had been discovered by eye doctors. The ancient Egyptians washed purulent eyes with urine, laid compresses on sties, and were convinced that a continuous wetting of the eyes with urine would prolong the eyes' visual acuity.

The founder of Western medicine (Hippocrates 460–377 B.C.), was the next to write about his explorations with the healing possibilities of urine. In his records he describes "Uropoty" as a remedy for the first time, the drinking of one's own urine.

In Japan urine therapy has been known for seven hundred years and is commonly prescribed even today against asthma, diabetes, and hypertension, and on an experimental basis against AIDS and cancer.

In Germany urine treatments have been used since medieval times against all kinds of diseases. Basically, almost every generation up to the present day has known urine as a miracle cure. Only in the last fifty years (without the experience of war and the postwar hardships) has the belief in pharmaceuticals, which have become readily available everywhere, pushed many natural remedies out of our consciousness. However, since the publication of my first urine therapy book I've received lots of letters confirming that many people today are taking another look at the old healing methods and are often more open to urine therapy than would be expected.

In India urine applications of a medical nature were first mentioned in the scripts of the *Bhava-mishra* (sixteenth century) and knowledge about the healing power of urine is widespread even today.

The Chinese were the first to associate a psychological effect with urine. They thought that the drinking of urine would strengthen their self-esteem and give them control over fear.

OTHER BENEFITS
OF URINE

Traditionally, hides, skins, and leather have been placed in urine for curing. In this way the material becomes smooth and possible parasites are killed. Afterward, the pieces must be rinsed with water; if this isn't done thoroughly the leather will smell like ammonia. To pee into your shoes makes the leather soft and pliable, as was well known to soldiers of all times. In this way they managed to prevent their feet from rubbing painfully in stiff boots during their long miles of marching.

Also, before chemical dyes, colorfast material could only be obtained by soaking the cloth in a urine bath after coloring it. For this the urine of an entire town was sometimes collected. After the First and Second World Wars many people in Germany remembered this old technique. In many countries in the third world material is still dyed in this way.

On a Greek island that did not have a spring and was dependent on water-tank boats, a vacationing woman made the discovery that her landlady cleaned her rented apartment with the urine of her children.

Nothing cleaned the tiles better, the native woman told her. An astonishing side effect: The flies avoided the house.

Berber tribes in the desert use camel urine to clean their dishes. And many tourists, who learn to honor the value of water when they drive through the desert, know how clean and free of grease car windows can get when washed with urine.

Karl May, a famous German writer, discovered an invisible ink—urine. Once the yellow liquid has dried, it cannot be seen anymore. Only if the recipient holds the letter over a hot stove plate, to warm the paper, can the writing be read.

And many flower gardeners, praised for their green thumbs, will tell you behind closed doors that a 1:1 solution of water and urine is responsible for their plants' flowering beauty.

Urine could be a versatile all-around tool if we could just learn to throw our artificially constructed inhibitions overboard. The possibilities for using urine are almost endless. Trying it out is better than just studying it!